Patient-Reported Outcomes in Endocrine Diseases

Editor

ELIZA B. GEER

ENDOCRINOLOGY AND METABOLISM CLINICS OF NORTH AMERICA

www.endo.theclinics.com

Consulting Editor

ADRIANA G. IOACHIMESCU

December 2022 • Volume 51 • Number 4

ELSEVIER

1600 John F. Kennedy Boulevard • Suite 1800 • Philadelphia, Pennsylvania, 19103-2899

http://www.theclinics.com

ENDOCRINOLOGY AND METABOLISM CLINICS OF NORTH AMERICA Volume 51, Number 4
December 2022 ISSN 0889-8529, ISBN 13: 978-0-323-96153-0

Editor: Katerina Heidhausen
Developmental Editor: Jessica Cañaberal

Endocrinology and Metabolism Clinics of North America (ISSN 0889-8529) is published quarterly by Elsevier Inc., 360 Park Avenue South, New York, NY 10010-1710. Months of issue are March, June, September, and December. Periodicals postage paid at New York, NY and additional mailing offices. Subscription prices are USD 394.00 per year for US individuals, USD 1058.00 per year for US institutions, USD 100.00 per year for US students and residents, USD 467.00 per year for Canadian individuals, USD 1079.00 per year for Canadian institutions, USD 512.00 per year for international individuals, USD 1079.00 per year for international institutions, USD 100.00 per year for Canadian students/residents, and USD 245.00 per year for international students/residents. To receive student/resident rate, orders must be accompanied by name of affiliated institution, date of term, and the signature of program/residency coordinator on institution letterhead. Orders will be billed at individual rate until proof of status is received. Foreign air speed delivery is included in all *Clinics* subscription prices All prices are subject to change without notice. **POSTMASTER:** Send address changes to *Endocrinology and Metabolism Clinics of North America*, Elsevier Health Sciences Division, Subscription Customer Service, 3251 Riverport Lane, Maryland Heights, MO 63043. **Customer Service: Telephone: 1-800-654-2452** (U.S. and Canada); **1-314-447-8871** (outside U.S. and Canada). **Fax: 1-314-447-8029. E-mail: journalscustomerservice-usa@elsevier.com (for print support)**; **journalsonlinesupport-usa@elsevier.com (for online support)**.

Reprints. For copies of 100 or more, of articles in this publication, please contact the Commercial Rights Department, Elsevier Inc., 360 Park Avenue South, New York, NY 10010-1710; phone: +1-212-633-3874 fax: +1-212-633-3820; E-mail: reprints@elsevier.com.

Endocrinology and Metabolism Clinics of North America is covered in *MEDLINE/PubMed (Index Medicus), EMBASE/Excerpta Medica, Current Contents/Clinical Medicine, Current Contents/Life Sciences, Science Citation Index, ISI/BIOMED, BIOSIS,* and *Chemical Abstracts*.

Contributors

CONSULTING EDITOR

ADRIANA G. IOACHIMESCU, MD, PhD, FACE
Professor, Departments of Medicine, Endocrinology and Metabolism, and Neurosurgery, Emory University School of Medicine, Atlanta, Georgia, USA

EDITOR

ELIZA B. GEER, MD
Medical Director, Multidisciplinary Pituitary and Skull Base Tumor Center, Associate Attending, Endocrinology Service, Departments of Medicine and Neurosurgery, Memorial Sloan Kettering Cancer Center, David H. Koch Center for Cancer Care, New York, New York, USA

AUTHORS

ZAKI ABOU-MRAD, MD
Department of Neurosurgery, Pituitary and Skull Base Tumor Program, Memorial Sloan Kettering Cancer Center, New York, New York, USA

CORNELIE D. ANDELA, MD, PhD
Department of Medicine, Division of Endocrinology, Center for Endocrine Tumors Leiden (CETL), Center for Pituitary Care, Leiden University Medical Center, Leiden, the Netherlands; Basalt Rehabilitation Center, The Hague, the Netherlands

CAROLINE APOVIAN, MD, FACP, FTOS, DABOM
Division of Endocrinology, Diabetes and Hypertension, Professor of Medicine and Pediatrics, Co-Director, Center for Weight Management and Wellness, Division of Endocrinology, Diabetes and Hypertension, Brigham and Women's Hospital, Boston, Massachusetts, USA

NIENKE R. BIERMASZ, MD, PhD
Department of Medicine, Division of Endocrinology, Center for Endocrine Tumors Leiden (CETL), Center for Pituitary Care, Leiden University Medical Center, Leiden, the Netherlands

RABIH BOU-NASSIF, MD
Department of Neurosurgery, Pituitary and Skull Base Tumor Program, Memorial Sloan Kettering Cancer Center, New York, New York, USA

CHRISTOPH BUETTNER, MD, PhD
Division Chief, Professor of Medicine, Chancellor-Scholar, Vice Chair of Basic Research, Department of Medicine, Division of Endocrinology, Metabolism and Nutrition, Rutgers, The State University of New Jersey, New Brunswick, New Jersey, USA

KHADEEN CHRISTI CHEESMAN, MD
Division of Endocrinology, Diabetes, and Bone Diseases, Department of Medicine, Icahn School of Medicine at Mount Sinai, New York, New York, USA

LUISELLA CIANFEROTTI, MD, PhD
Department of Experimental and Clinical Biomedical Sciences "Mario Serio," University of Florence, Florence, Italy

CRISTIANA CIPRIANI, MD, PhD
Department of Clinical, Internal, Anesthesiological and Cardiovascular Sciences, Sapienza University of Rome, Rome, Italy

KIM M.J.A. CLAESSEN, MD, PhD
Department of Medicine, Division of Endocrinology, Center for Endocrine Tumors Leiden (CETL), Center for Pituitary Care, Leiden University Medical Center, Leiden, the Netherlands

MARC A. COHEN, MD
Pituitary and Skull Base Tumor Program, Head and Neck Service, Department of Surgery, Memorial Sloan Kettering Cancer Center, New York, New York, USA

EVA C. COOPMANS, MD, PhD
Department of Medicine, Division of Endocrinology, Center for Endocrine Tumors Leiden (CETL), Center for Pituitary Care, Leiden University Medical Center, Leiden, the Netherlands

TAREK Y. EL AHMADIEH, MD
Department of Neurosurgery, Pituitary and Skull Base Tumor Program, Memorial Sloan Kettering Cancer Center, New York, New York, USA

ELIZA B. GEER, MD
Medical Director, Multidisciplinary Pituitary and Skull Base Tumor Center, Associate Attending, Endocrinology Service, Departments of Medicine and Neurosurgery, Memorial Sloan Kettering Cancer Center, David H. Koch Center for Cancer Care, New York, New York, USA

NAMRATA GUMASTE, MD
Department of Medicine, Weill Cornell Medicine, NewYork-Presbyterian Hospital, New York, New York, USA

SAMAR HAFIDA, MD
Assistant Professor, Boston University School of Medicine, Division of Endocrinology, Diabetes, Nutrition and Weight Management, Boston, Massachusetts, USA

MARTHA HICKEY, MBChB, MD
Department of Obstetrics and Gynaecology, University of Melbourne, The Royal Women's Hospital, Melbourne, Victoria, Australia

HYON KIM, MD
Assistant Professor, Department of Medicine, Division of Endocrinology, Metabolism and Nutrition, Rutgers, The State University of New Jersey, New Brunswick, New Jersey, USA

BENITA KNOX, MD
The Royal Women's Hospital, Melbourne, Victoria, Australia

DINGFENG LI, MD, MSc
Assistant Professor of Medicine, Department of Endocrinology, Endocrine and Metabolism Institute, Cleveland Clinic, Cleveland, Ohio, USA

SUSAN C. PITT, MD, MPHS
Associate Professor, Department of Surgery, University of Michigan, Ann Arbor, Michigan, USA

KUNAL SHAH, MD
Assistant Professor, Department of Medicine, Division of Endocrinology, Metabolism and Nutrition, Rutgers, The State University of New Jersey, New Brunswick, New Jersey, USA

LEENA SHAH, MD
Division of Endocrinology, Diabetes, and Bone Diseases, Department of Medicine, Icahn School of Medicine at Mount Sinai, New York, New York, USA

PETER J. SNYDER, MD
Professor of Medicine, Division of Endocrinology, Diabetes and Metabolism, Perelman School of Medicine, University of Pennsylvania, Philadelphia, Pennsylvania, USA

CORD STURGEON, MD, MS
Professor, Department of Surgery, Northwestern University, Chicago, Illinois, USA

VIVIANE TABAR, MD
Department of Neurosurgery, Pituitary and Skull Base Tumor Program, Memorial Sloan Kettering Cancer Center, New York, New York, USA

LOUIE YE, MD, PhD
Department of Obstetrics and Gynaecology, University of Melbourne, The Royal Women's Hospital, Melbourne, Victoria, Australia

KYLE ZANOCCO, MD, MS
Assistant Professor, Department of Surgery, University of California, Los Angeles, Los Angeles, California, USA

Contents

Foreword: Importance of Patient-Reported Outcomes in Endocrinology xi

Adriana G. Ioachimescu

Preface: Patient-Reported Outcomes in Endocrinology xv

Eliza B. Geer

Evaluating Patient-Reported Outcomes in Cushing's Syndrome 691

Namrata Gumaste, Leena Shah, Khadeen Christi Cheesman, and Eliza B. Geer

The importance of the patient's perspective on disease has increasingly gained traction among clinical investigators and clinicians. Patient-reported outcomes (PROs) are those which pertain to a patient's health, quality of life, or functional status (associated with health care or treatment) that are reported directly by the patient, without interpretation by a clinician. In this article, we will review PROs as they relate to the signs, symptoms, health-related quality of life, and comorbidities of active Cushing's syndrome (CS), and CS after treatment with surgery, radiotherapy, and medical therapy. We will explore long-term outcomes in the setting of remission, persistence, and recurrence in this population.

Evaluating the Impact of Acromegaly on Quality of Life 709

Eva C. Coopmans, Cornelie D. Andela, Kim M.J.A. Claessen, and Nienke R. Biermasz

Acromegaly has a substantial negative impact on quality of life (QoL). This review aims to discuss the impact of acromegaly on QoL from the clinical perspective as well as from the patient perspective. Furthermore, it aims to evaluate the use of patient-reported outcome measures (PROMs) in acromegaly and how PROMs aid decision-making. The recommendations presented in this review are based on recent clinical evidence on the impact of acromegaly on QoL combined with the authors' own clinical experience treating patients with acromegaly. We recommend that a patient-centered approach should be considered in treatment decisions, integrating conventional biochemical outcomes, tumor control, comorbidities, treatment complications, and PROMs, including QoL measures. This more integrated approach seems effective in treating comorbidities and improving patient-reported outcomes and is critical, as many patients do not achieve biochemical or tumor control and comorbidities, impairment in QoL may not remit even when full biochemical control is achieved.

Patient-Reported Outcomes in Endoscopic Endonasal Skull Base Surgery 727

Rabih Bou-Nassif, Zaki Abou-Mrad, Tarek Y. El Ahmadieh, Viviane Tabar, and Marc A. Cohen

The functional outcome, quality of life, and patient feedback related to a chosen treatment approach in skull base surgery have become a subject of interest and focused research in recent years. The current advances in endoscopic optical imaging technology and surgical precision have radically lowered the perioperative morbidity associated with skull base surgery. This has pushed toward a higher focus on patient-reported outcomes (PROs). It is now critical to ensure that the offered treatment plan and approach align with the patient's preferences and expectations, in addition to the surgeon's best clinical judgment and experience. PROs represent a view that reflects the patient's own thoughts and perspective on their condition and the management options, without input or interpretations from the surgeon. Having PRO data enables patients the opportunity to learn from the experiences and perspectives of other patients. This input empowers the patient to become an active participant in the decision-making process at different stages of their care. An in-depth PRO evaluation requires specific validated tools and scoring systems, namely the patient-reported outcomes measures (PROM) tools. In this review, we discuss the currently available skull-base-related PROs, the assessment tools used to capture them, and the future trends of this important topic that is in its infancy.

Quality of Life in Patients with Adrenal Insufficiency **741**

Dingfeng Li

Patients with adrenal insufficiency, despite standard glucocorticoid replacement therapy, continue to experience and report impaired self-perceived health status and quality of life. In this review, we will describe quality of life in this patient population, and summarize the determinants of quality of life, based on previous survey-based studies and clinical trials. In addition, some new emerging data during the still ongoing coronavirus disease pandemic are also reviewed in the present article.

Symptoms of Late-Onset Hypogonadism in Men **755**

Peter J. Snyder

A small percentage of older men are hypogonadal for no apparent reason other than age, a condition called late-onset hypogonadism. This condition is accompanied by symptoms, especially sexual symptoms, most notably decreased libido. Testosterone treatment of men who have late-onset hypogonadism improves all aspects of sexual function and also mood, depressive symptoms, and self-reported walking ability. Testosterone treatment would not be expected to improve similar symptoms in men who are not unequivocally hypogonadal.

The Patient Experience of Thyroid Cancer **761**

Susan C. Pitt, Kyle Zanocco, and Cord Sturgeon

The 3 phases of thyroid cancer care are discussed: diagnosis, management, and survivorship. Drivers of quality of life (QOL) in each phase are described, and suggestions are made for mitigating the risk of poor QOL. Active surveillance is another emerging management strategy that has the potential to improve QOL by eliminating upfront surgical morbidity but will need to be studied prospectively.

Use of Patient-Reported Outcomes for Assessing Diabetes Outcomes **781**

Hyon Kim, Kunal Shah, and Christoph Buettner

The treatment of diabetes can be complex and overwhelming for patients as it demands persistent attention to lifestyle management, adherence to medications, monitoring of side effects of drugs, and management of devices for glucose monitoring and/or insulin infusion. Therefore, understanding patient-reported outcomes (PROs) that provide direct insight into the patient's experience with diabetes is crucial for optimizing diabetes management.This review provides an overview of commonly used PRO questionnaires that assess different aspects of diabetes management.

Physiology of the Weight-Reduced State and Its Impact on Weight Regain **795**

Samar Hafida and Caroline Apovian

Obesity is a chronic disease characterized by long duration, slow progression, and periods of remission and relapses. Despite the development of effective medical and surgical interventions and millions of people conducting tremendous personal efforts to manage their weight every year, recidivism remains a significant barrier to attaining long-term weight maintenance. This review aimed to explain the underlying physiology of the weight-reduced state including changes in energy balance, adipose tissue, genetic, environmental, and behavioral factors that may predispose individuals to weight regain following weight loss.

Management of Menopause Symptoms and Quality of Life during the Menopause Transition **817**

Louie Ye, Benita Knox, and Martha Hickey

Some women experience bothersome symptoms around the time of menopause that may have a negative impact on their quality of life and prompt them to seek treatments. Menopausal hormone therapy was historically the treatment of choice. However, medical contraindications and personal preference for nonhormonal therapy have prompted the evaluation of a range of nonhormonal pharmacologic and non-pharmacologic therapies. This review provides an update focusing on the latest evidence-based approach for the management of bothersome symptoms of menopause.

Quality of Life in Primary Hyperparathyroidism **837**

Cristiana Cipriani and Luisella Cianferotti

Quality of life is impaired in primary hyperparathyroidism (PHPT), regardless of the severity of the disease. Clinical studies have employed different instruments, including standardized and disease-specific questionnaires, and including patients with different phenotypes of PHPT. Neuropsychiatric symptoms and decline in cognitive status are common in PHPT. Patients may complain of these issues or they can be ascertained by questionnaires; they include depression, anxiety, impaired vitality, social and emotional functions, sleep disturbances, and altered mental function. Randomized controlled trials on the effects of surgical versus non-surgical treatments have collectively shown improvement in quality of life after parathyroidectomy, but results have been heterogeneous.

ENDOCRINOLOGY AND METABOLISM CLINICS OF NORTH AMERICA

FORTHCOMING ISSUES

March 2023
Diabetes Remission
Betul Hatipoglu, *Editor*

June 2023
Endocrinology of the Aging Patient
Rita Rastogi Kalyani, *Editor*

September 2023
Metabolic Associated Fatty Liver Disease
Sherouk Fouda and Joseph M. Pappachan, *Editors*

RECENT ISSUES

September 2022
Lipids: Update on Diagnosis and Management of Dyslipidemia
Connie B. Newman and Alan Chait, *Editors*

June 2022
Updates in Thyroidology
Megan Haymart and Maria Papaleontiou, *Editors*

March 2022
Hypogonadism
Shalender Bhasin and Channa Jayasena, *Editors*

SERIES OF RELATED INTEREST

Medical Clinics
https://www.medical.theclinics.com
Primary Care: Clinics in Office Practice
https://www.primarycare.theclinics.com/

Foreword
Importance of Patient-Reported Outcomes in Endocrinology

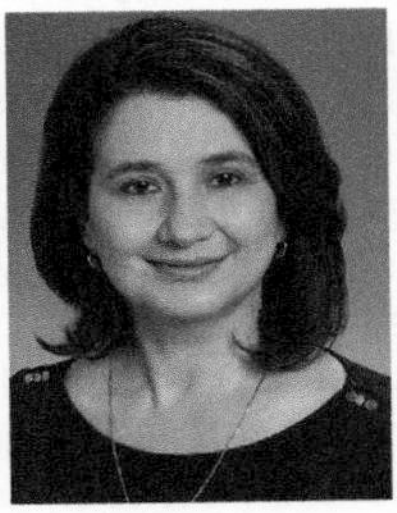

Adriana G. Ioachimescu, MD, PhD, FACE
Consulting Editor

We dedicate the current issue of the *Endocrinology and Metabolism Clinics of North America* to patient-reported outcomes (PROs), an emerging field in health care delivery and research. Patients' perception about health and disease, including their quality of life (QoL) and the effects of treatment on their functional status, can be evaluated with general and disease-specific parameter instruments. Implementation of the PROs in the management of various endocrine disorder is currently unfolding and offers opportunities for improved patient-clinician communication, education, and research. The process entails PRO validation and interpretation in context of the conventional outcomes used by clinicians (for example, normalization of hormone levels), design of a patient-centric management plan, and a greater involvement of patients in the decision making.

The guest editor of this issue is Dr Eliza B. Geer, the medical director of the Multidisciplinary Pituitary and Skull Base Tumor Center from Memorial Sloan Kettering Cancer Center in New York. Dr Geer is a well-known expert in PRO in acromegaly and Cushing syndrome. The issue includes 10 articles, which address pathologic condition of the adrenal, pituitary, thyroid, parathyroid and gonadal glands, as well as diabetes and obesity.

The effects of active hypercortisolism on multiple organs and systems are both acute and chronic. The use of PROs in patients with endogenous Cushing syndrome has unveiled its long-lasting consequences on QoL, functional status, and mental health, even in patients who achieved biochemical remission. Some comorbidities may persist after remission (including hypopituitarism, obesity, depression) and require lifelong specific treatment. PRO research is needed to understand the effects of medical and radiation treatment on patients with persistent or recurrent hypercortisolism postoperatively.

Endocrinol Metab Clin N Am 51 (2022) xi–xiii
https://doi.org/10.1016/j.ecl.2022.06.008
0889-8529/22/© 2022 Published by Elsevier Inc.

In patients with adrenal insufficiency, QoL is lower compared with the general population despite glucocorticoid replacement therapy. Older age, sex (female for Addison disease), and type of adrenal insufficiency (secondary and glucocorticoid-induced worse than primary), as well as insufficient family support and higher financial burden were associated with worse QoL scores. Patient education, supportive social and financial measures, as well as modification of glucocorticoid replacement strategies are recommended.

The consequences of excess growth hormone in patients with acromegaly include a large array of symptoms, physical deformities, and comorbidities. Unfortunately, due to insidious onset and delayed diagnosis of acromegaly, some problems persist after treatment, even when biochemical normalization and tumor removal or control were achieved. In particular, musculoskeletal burden of disease can worsen with age. Also, PROs are important for those patients with discordant insulin-like growth factor-1 and growth hormone levels and can guide the next steps of treatment.

For patients with sellar and suprasellar masses, tools have been developed to address endoscopic surgery outcomes, such as olfactory dysfunction, sinonasal complications, and visual and functional changes. A collaboration between neurosurgery and otolaryngology is essential for the first two problems.

QoL of thyroid cancer survivors is lower than in the general population. In part, this is related to direct consequences of surgery (hypothyroidism, possible injury of the recurrent laryngeal nerve, or hypoparathyroidism) or radioactive iodine therapy (sialadenitis). PRO research contributed to the changes in management over the years, including minimizing the extent of surgery, limiting the use of radioactive iodine, and implementation of active surveillance plans.

Primary hyperparathyroidism has been associated with QoL impairment in the physical, neurocognitive, mood, and functional domains. Overall, QoL has been shown to improve after parathyroid surgery. However, prospective and randomized controlled study did not show a consistent long-term improvement of neuropsychiatric and cognitive function postoperatively.

Menopause associates multiple symptoms, including vasomotor, urogenital, sleep, cognitive, and mood disturbances, which all impact the QoL. Several pharmacologic (hormonal and nonhormonal) and nonpharmacologic options exist, which require optimization and future study.

Late-onset hypogonadism in men is defined as aging-related symptomatic hypogonadism without another identifiable cause. These patients may have sexual dysfunction, depressed moods, decreased energy, and functional changes (walking ability). PRO research indicated that self-reported sexual function usually ameliorates with testosterone replacement, while other manifestations improve to a smaller degree.

Diabetes research found that PROs are useful tools to identify factors of medication and dietary adherence, as well as treatment side effects. In recent years, technological advances have expanded the array of treatment choices and increased patients' involvement in medical decisions. Some diabetes medications have been shown to improve patient satisfaction. It is important to know that clinician-determined outcomes do not always correlate with PROs, which require additional investigation, such as screening for depression or fear of hypoglycemia.

Obesity is a chronic condition, with most patients experiencing weight regain after successful weight loss, which has been associated with impaired QoL. PRO research can guide strategies to anticipate and mitigate weight regain, which are based on genetic, personality, cultural, and environmental factors.

I hope you will find this issue of the *Endocrinology and Metabolism Clinics of North America* informative and helpful in your practice. I thank Dr Geer for guest-editing this important issue and the authors for their work. I thank the Elsevier editorial staff for their constant support.

Adriana G. Ioachimescu, MD, PhD, FACE
Departments of Medicine, Endocrinology and Metabolism, and Neurosurgery
Emory University School of Medicine
1365 B Clifton Road, Northeast, B6209
Atlanta, GA 30322, USA

E-mail address:
aioachi@emory.edu

Preface
Patient-Reported Outcomes in Endocrinology

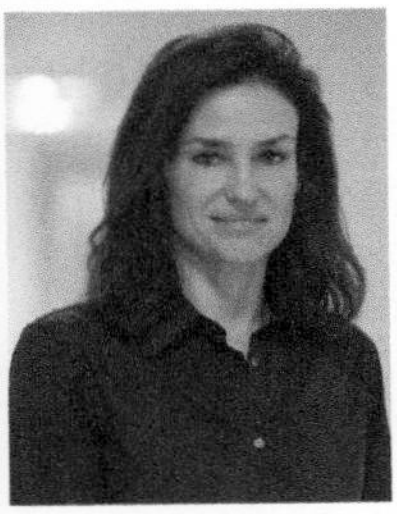

Eliza B. Geer, MD
Editor

The importance of the patient's perspective on disease has recently gained salience among clinical investigators and clinicians. Patient-reported outcomes (PROs) are those that pertain to a patient's health, quality if life, or functional status, that are associated with health care or treatment, and reported directly by the patient, without interpretation by a clinician. In any condition, PROs are critical tools to assess disease severity and the benefits and risks of a given treatment. Disease-specific, generic, and symptom-specific assessments each contribute valuable perspectives on the short- and long-term burden of the medical condition and its treatment from a patient's perspective. This issue of *Endocrinology and Metabolism Clinics of North America* includes a series of articles that review the use of PROs in a range of endocrine diseases.

Practitioners managing endocrine conditions, whether diabetes, thyroid cancer, Cushing, or acromegaly, typically focus on normalizing hormone levels, achieving stability on imaging, and preventing tumor growth, if applicable. These are critical outcomes that need to be addressed. But we also need to focus on the patient's perspective and ask more questions. Have our treatments been successful if the patient is still symptomatic despite achieving endocrine remission? Do we define remission/treatment success based on circulating hormone concentrations and imaging alone, or do we also include "remission" of disease-specific PROs? Do clinical trials investigating new therapies adequately include PROs in order to assess treatment outcomes? We need to critically assess the conventional outcomes and treatment goals that have been historically used and engage our patients to share their story. The more we solicit our patients' treatment goals and priorities, the more we will start to ask the right questions. These questions in turn will allow clinicians and investigators to identify the best answers (ie, the right treatments) to address our patients' suffering.

Functional remission, which is clinical remission plus recovery of daily functioning in the social, professional, and personal domains, is the ultimate goal for our patients. In

Endocrinol Metab Clin N Am 51 (2022) xv–xvi
https://doi.org/10.1016/j.ecl.2022.06.001

order to achieve this, an accurate and thorough understanding of how patients experience their diagnosis, treatment effects, and associated comorbidities is essential. Further research is needed to assess and develop critical PROs for endocrine patients receiving long-term medical treatment. This will help guide the direction of ongoing and future medical therapy development with a critical focus on therapies that address the ongoing symptom burden that many patients experience despite successful treatment. Ultimately, consistent and appropriate use of validated PROs will lead to the development of therapies that not only address objective disease-specific metrics but also address the subjective patient experience.

Eliza B. Geer, MD
Multidisciplinary Pituitary and
Skull Base Tumor Center
Endocrinology Service
Departments of Medicine and Neurosurgery
Memorial Sloan Kettering Cancer Center
David H. Koch Center for Cancer Care
530 East 74th Street, Box 19
New York, NY 10021, USA

E-mail address:
geere@mskcc.org

Evaluating Patient-Reported Outcomes in Cushing's Syndrome

Namrata Gumaste, MD[a], Leena Shah, MD[b],
Khadeen Christi Cheesman, MD[b], Eliza B. Geer, MD[c,d,*]

KEYWORDS

- Cushing's syndrome • Cushing's disease • Patient-reported outcomes
- Quality of life

KEY POINTS

- Patients with active CS experience a wide range of signs and symptoms, and notably report impaired health-related quality of life when compared with those who have achieved biochemical remission and normative controls.
- Medical therapy for CS is emerging as a more viable option for disease control for patients with recurrent disease after surgery or who are not surgical candidates, with some studies showing improvement in patient-reported outcomes (PROs) with medical management.
- Impaired health-related quality of life can persist even after successful surgery in Cushing's syndrome in part because comorbidities due to chronic hypercortisolemia may persist long after surgical remission. It is essential to perform periodic, life-long evaluations to properly manage persistent comorbidities after surgery.
- Patient-reported outcomes are affected by hypopituitarism and delay in effect in patients with Cushing's disease who are treated with radiotherapy.
- Impaired health-related quality of life may persist in patients with Cushing's syndrome even after long-term treatment, possibly due to the persistent effects of prior excess cortisol exposure, or differences in the definitions of Cushing's remission resulting in heterogeneity in remitted cohorts.

[a] Department of Medicine, Weill Cornell Medicine, New York-Presbyterian Hospital, 505 East 70th Street, Suite 450, New York, NY 10021, USA; [b] Division of Endocrinology, Diabetes, and Bone Diseases, Department of Medicine, Icahn School of Medicine at Mount Sinai, One Gustave L Levy Place, Box 1055, New York, NY 10029, USA; [c] Department of Medicine, Multidisciplinary Pituitary and Skull Base Tumor Center, Memorial Sloan Kettering Cancer Center, David H. Koch Center for Cancer Care, 530 East 74th Street, Box 19, New York, NY 10021, USA; [d] Department of Neurosurgery, Multidisciplinary Pituitary and Skull Base Tumor Center, Memorial Sloan Kettering Cancer Center, David H. Koch Center for Cancer Care, 530 East 74th Street, Box 19, New York, NY 10021, USA
* Corresponding author. Memorial Sloan Kettering Cancer Center, David H. Koch Center for Cancer Care, 530 East Street 74th Street, Box 19, New York, NY 10021.
E-mail address: geere@mskcc.org

Endocrinol Metab Clin N Am 51 (2022) 691–707
https://doi.org/10.1016/j.ecl.2022.05.002

INTRODUCTION

Endogenous Cushing's syndrome (CS) is a rare hormonal disorder with an annual incidence of 1.8 to 3.2 persons per million.[1] It is defined by the body's prolonged exposure to excess cortisol, caused primarily from ACTH-secreting pituitary adenomas (Cushing's disease, CD), cortisol-secreting adrenal adenomas or ectopic ACTH-secreting tumors.[2] Rare diseases such as CS often leave patients alienated, as there are limited health care providers and centers able to deliver specialized care. In recent decades, the importance of the patient's perspective on disease has increasingly gained traction among clinical investigators and clinicians.[2] Patient-reported outcomes (PROs) are those which pertain to a patient's health, quality of life, or functional status (associated with health care or treatment) that are reported directly by the patient, without interpretation by a clinician.[3] In this article, we will review PROs as they relate to the signs, symptoms, and comorbidities of active CS, and CS after treatment with medication, surgery, and radiotherapy. We will explore long-term outcomes in the setting of remission, persistence, and recurrence in this population.

SYMPTOMS, SIGNS, AND COMORBIDITIES IN ACTIVE CUSHING'S SYNDROME

The signs and symptoms of overt hypercortisolism are well known; however, the presentation of CS can vary greatly. Common presentations include weight gain, decreased libido, plethora, round face, dorsal fat pad, menstrual changes, hirsutism, edema, proximal muscle weakness, hypertension, bruising, depression, and lethargy.[4] Patients with CS suffer from a multitude of comorbid conditions, such as cardiovascular (atherosclerosis, left ventricular hypertrophy, systolic and diastolic dysfunction), metabolic (dyslipidemia, central obesity, diabetes mellitus (DM)), thrombotic disorders, bone disorders (osteoporosis), immune deficits, and cognitive and neuropsychological impairment.[5]

The European Registry on Cushing Syndrome (ERCUSYN) is a large database that was designed to prospectively collect data on patients with CS.[6] All sign and symptom data were generated from patient input into the database. A total of 481 patients were analyzed in the initial database publication, 19% of whom were men, and with an average age of 44.2 years at diagnosis. The most common signs and symptoms reported in the registry at diagnosis included weight gain, hypertension, skin alterations, myopathy, hirsutism, menstrual irregularities, reduced libido, depression, diabetes mellitus, hair loss, and bone fractures. Of these clinical features, the most prevalent at diagnosis were weight gain (81%), hypertension (78%), skin alternations (73%), and myopathy (67%). There were differences in the prevalence of symptoms based on CS etiology, with a higher rate of hirsutism in female patients with ectopic CS compared with other etiologies. DM was more prevalent in patients with ectopic CS. Patients with pituitary CS had more skin alterations, menstrual irregularities, and hirsutism compared with those with adrenal CS. Weight gain (86%), hypertension (77%), and myopathy (66%) were most prevalent among women. In men, hypertension (83%), myopathy (71%), and reduced libido (69%) were most common.

In a pilot study by Webb and colleagues, a structured interview was used to elicit symptoms in patients with pituitary and parasellar diseases and how these impacted their daily lives.[7] Fifty-four patients were interviewed, of which 14 had CD. Patients were asked about physical changes observed at diagnosis and later after treatment. At diagnosis, patients reported swelling, weight gain, excessive fatigability, change in body shape, hirsutism, pain, bruising, difficulty sleeping, and menstrual irregularities.[7] Depression, irritability, mood swings, and anxiety, were also reported at diagnosis, though emotional symptoms were not separated by pituitary disease type.

Overall, patients with CD reported that their disease had the greatest impact on their lives (7.5 on a maximum scale of 10), compared with patients with other pituitary tumors (6.5 for acromegaly, 6.8 for prolactinoma, and 5.8 for nonfunctioning adenomas).

Patients with active CS demonstrate psychiatric and neurocognitive impairments including depression, anxiety, mania, insomnia, issues with memory, concentration, visuospatial functioning, and language functioning.[8] Depression is the most common psychiatric comorbidity described in CS, and studies show that a diagnosis of major depressive disorder occurs in 50% to 80% of patients with active disease.[9] In the first prospective study by Starkman and colleagues describing neuropsychiatric symptoms in CS, patients reported increased crying (63%), suicidal thoughts (17%), suicide attempts (5%), and social withdrawal (46%).[9] Anxiety is another commonly reported symptom. In one older study by Loosen and colleagues, DSM-III-R criteria were used to evaluate patients and showed a prevalence of 79% for generalized anxiety disorder in this population.[10] In 2 other studies without specific diagnostic criteria, anxiety was reported in 66%[9] of patients in active disease, and pathologic anxiety in 12%.[11] In a study by Santos and colleagues, patients with active CS had worse depression and anxiety scores compared with controls, as rated using the Beck's Depression Inventory (BDI) questionnaire and the State-Trait Anxiety Index (STAI), respectively.[12]

Although the signs and symptoms of CS have been well documented, evidence is still lacking regarding how these clinical features directly correlate with health-related quality of life (HRQoL).[13] A clinical trial investigating pasireotide treatment in patients with CD did not identify a statistically significant difference in HRQoL based on the severity of signs and symptoms such as bruising, rubor, or fat deposition at baseline and after treatment.[14,15] This study was limited by baseline mild symptom severity in the cohort, and a small sample size (N = 78) that completed the 12 month trial.[14,15] To date, depression is the only symptom that has been shown to directly impact HRQoL.[6,14] It is clear that signs and symptoms of CS affect patient HRQoL, as these are incorporated in all disease-specific HRQoL measures. The inability to identify a direct correlation of these signs and symptoms with HRQoL is more likely due to the lack of data and methodological difficulties proving causation.

HEALTH-RELATED QUALITY OF LIFE IN ACTIVE CUSHING'S SYNDROME

Given the symptom and comorbidity burden as described above, patients with CS experience impaired HRQoL. The CushingQoL and Tuebingen CD-25 are 2 disease-specific PRO measures that have been used in patients with CS, in addition to generic HRQoL measures, such as Short Form (SF)-36 and SF-12, and symptom-specific measures such as the Hospital Anxiety and Depression Scale (HADS), BDI, and the Multidimensional Fatigue Inventory (MFI).[16] **Table 1** includes a list of PRO questionnaires that have been used in patients with CS.[17–27]

CushingQoL

The CushingQoL was the first Cushing-specific questionnaire designed by Webb and colleagues to asses HRQoL in CS.[28] The 12 item questionnaire is self-administered and includes the following domains: difficulty sleeping, wound healing/bruising, irritability/mood swings/anger, self-confidence, physical changes, ability to participate in activities, interactions with friends/family, memory issues, and future health concerns.[13] Each question has 5 response categories that are rated on a scale of 1 to 5, with 1 corresponding to "always" or "very much" and 5 corresponding to "never" or "not at all." Ten patients with CS were interviewed regarding how CS had affected

Table 1
Review of select validated PRO questionnaires

Patient-Reported Outcome Assessments[17]	Normative Data Available?	Number of CS Studies Using Assessment	Scoring (Clinical Cutoff or Minimal Important Difference, if Available)
Generic QoL Assessments			
Notingham Health Profile (NHP)	No	2	Score 0–100, higher score = worse QoL[18]
Short Form-36 (SF-36)	Yes	23	Score 0–100, higher score = better QoL[18] (5-point minimal detectable change in a normative sample[18])
Short Form-12 (SF-12) (abbreviated version of SF-36)	Yes	1	Score 0–100, higher score = better QoL[18]
World Health Organization Quality of Life BREF (WHOQoL-BREF)	Yes	5	Score 0–100, higher score = better QoL[19]
Cushing Specific QoL Assessments			
CushingQoL	No	25	Score 12–60, higher score = better QoL, can be standardized on 0–100 scale[20] (10.1 point difference, minimal important difference[20])
Tuebingen CD-25	Yes	7	Score 0–100, higher score = worse QoL[21]
Symptom Specific Assessments			
State Trait Anxiety Inventory (STAI)	Yes	6	Score 20–80, higher score = greater anxiety[22] (Total score 39–40 cutoff for clinically significant anxiety, 54–55 suggested in older adults[22])
Hospital Anxiety and Depression Scale (HADS)	Yes	7	Score 0–21, higher score = greater symptoms of depression/anxiety[23]
Beck Depression Inventory-II (BDI-II)	Yes	15	Score 0–63, higher score = worse depression[24] (17.5% score reduction, minimal important difference, 32% in those with more severe depression[24])
Multidimensional Fatigue Inventory (MFI)	Yes	1	Score 4–20 per subscale, higher score = greater fatigue. Five subscales available, creators discourage the use of total score 20–100.[25]

(*continued on next page*)

Table 1
(*continued*)

Patient-Reported Outcome Assessments[17]	Normative Data Available?	Number of CS Studies Using Assessment	Scoring (Clinical Cutoff or Minimal Important Difference, if Available)
Female Sexual Function Index (FSFI)	Yes	1	Score 2–36, lower score = greater sexual dysfunction[26] (Total score <26.55 cutoff for sexual dysfunction[26])
Pittsburgh Sleep Quality Index (PSQI)	Yes	2	Score 0–21, higher score = worse sleep quality[27] (Total score >5 cutoff for poor sleep quality[27])

their lives to determine the domains. The validity and reliability of the CushingQoL were then investigated by Webb and colleagues in a multi-center cross-sectional study across 5 European countries. The study recruited 125 active and treated patients with CS (86% with CD and 14% with adrenal CS). Study participants were asked to complete the CushingQoL, the SF-36, and a single question on self-perceived general health. The CushingQoL was found to be a valid and reliable instrument, which was moderately correlated with all dimensions of the SF-36 (r between 0.3 and 0.7). Investigators found that active patients with CS reported worse QoL scores compared with those with controlled disease.[28] A later study determined the minimal important difference (MID) for the CushingQoL to be 10.1.[29,30] The MID provides a measure of the smallest change in a PRO that patients perceive as important.[31] In a longitudinal study by Santos and colleagues, which evaluated the test–retest reliability and sensitivity of the CushingQoL, patients with active disease were found to have significantly worse CushingQoL scores compared with those in remission.[32]

Tuebingen CD-25

The Tuebingen CD-25 is the second disease-specific questionnaire that was developed and validated for patients with CD. This distinguishes it from the CushingQoL, which was developed for pituitary and adrenal patients with CS. In a single-center cross-sectional retrospective study[21] 64 questions were generated using a threefold approach: the literature was reviewed, 10 patients with CD were interviewed regarding HRQoL factors, and endocrinologists, neurosurgeons, and neuropsychologists were asked to contribute regarding domains thought to impact patients with CD. Sixty-three patients with CD, including those with newly diagnosed CD and those after surgical resection, were given the 64-item questionnaire which included 6 domains: depression, sexual activity, environment, eating behavior, bodily restrictions, and cognition. The final version contained 25 items with these 6 subdomains. The questionnaire states "Because of my Cushing's disease..." and responses included a 5-point scale with 0 corresponding to "strongly disagree" and 4 corresponding to "strongly agree." Of the 63 patients recruited, 35 patients had undergone surgical resection but were asked to answer retrospectively. Of note, 10 of the 35 postoperative patients had recurrent CD. Patients were also asked to complete the abbreviated World Health Organization Quality of Life questionnaire (WHOQoL-BREF). Overall, the Tuebingen CD-25 was found to be valid and reliable, with moderate correlation (r = −0.65) between its total score and that of the WHOQoL-BREF. There was no correlation between preoperative plasma ACTH and serum cortisol levels and Tuebingen CD-25 scores in this study. However, 24-h mean urine free cortisol (mUFC) was significantly correlated with worse scores in the cognition subdomain, and almost met significance for the eating behavior subdomain.

After determining the validity and reliability of the Tuebingen CD-25, the authors aimed to assess normative data from healthy controls, which had not yet been conducted in a Cushing-specific PRO instrument. In this part of the study,[33] the Tuebingen CD-25 was administered to 1784 healthy controls from Germany via an online survey. The questionnaire was identical to the one administered to patients with CD, except the opening phrase was modified from "Because of my Cushing's disease..." to "In my daily life..." Compared with healthy controls, female patients with CD were found to have significant differences in all subscale scores and total Tuebingen CD-25 scores indicating impairment in HRQoL in this population. Although only 11 male patients with CD were enrolled in this study, significant differences were found in the bodily restriction and cognition subscales, compared with male healthy controls. Differences in the Tuebingen CD-25 total score between male patients with CD and healthy controls marginally failed significance; however, there was a trend toward worse HRQoL in this very small cohort of male patients with CD.

SURGICAL INTERVENTION IN CUSHING'S SYNDROME

Surgical resection of the disease-causing tumor is first-line treatment of CS.[34] However, comorbidities due to chronic hypercortisolemia may persist long after surgical remission, and consequently CS can be associated with impaired HRQoL even after successful surgery.[34] The timeline of postoperative improvement in symptoms varies and may take months to years.[17,34,35] Glucocorticoid withdrawal symptoms, which occur after successful surgery, can contribute to significant challenges and impaired HRQoL after surgery.[17]

Patient Perspectives After Surgical Resection

Patient-reported outcomes in patients with CS after surgery are affected by delayed symptom improvement and variation in symptom burden. A cross-sectional study of 91 surgically treated patients with CS (including 63 with CD who underwent transsphenoidal surgery (TSS) and 28 with adrenal CS who underwent unilateral adrenalectomy), found via self-reporting that patients do not consider surgical remission to be the same as recovery.[34] Patient responses to open-ended questions in this study highlighted the challenges in recovery.[34] All 91 patients self-reported that they had achieved surgical remission as defined by the reported need for cortisol replacement medication (CRM) postsurgery.[34] At the time of the survey, 25 of the 91 patients were still taking CRM and the patients who had discontinued CRM reported needing CRM for a median time of 10.5 months after surgery. Despite reporting surgical remission, 42 of the 91 patients (46%) indicated that they had not yet recovered, while 49 patients (54%) reported a median recovery time of 22 months after surgery. Recovery was not defined in the survey and was left to patient perception. Long duration of recovery was most frequently reported by patients, followed by pain and fatigue. Fifteen percent of patients also reported neuropsychiatric impairment (including memory loss, difficulty focusing, depression, anxiety, and mood changes) as a significant challenge to recovery.

In the same study, a second survey was developed based on the initial responses and given to a total of 341 patients with CS, who were considered to be in surgical remission based on either needing postoperative CRM or not needing any additional medications.

Patient responses were then compared with those of 54 endocrinologists.[34] Patients reported a median complete recovery time of 18 months, which was significantly longer than the perceived recovery time of 12 months reported by the endocrinologists. Patient-reported recovery time did not differ by CS etiology and exceeded CRM duration.[34] The need for CRM is often consistent with a successful surgical outcome, but patients may feel the need for medication reflects persistent disease.[36]

Health-Related Quality of Life After Surgical Resection

Validated questionnaires can help identify predictors for HRQoL in CS after surgery. A study by Santos and colleagues suggests that CushingQoL scores improve in the year after surgery.[32] The investigators asked 11 patients with active hypercortisolism to complete the CushingQoL before surgery (either TSS or adrenal surgery), and then 4 and 9 months postsurgery. Patients were confirmed to be biochemically cured, defined by the presence of adrenal insufficiency or the suppression of morning serum cortisol less than 50 nmol/L after 1 mg dexamethasone suppression test and a normal 24-h UFC. Compared with presurgery, CushingQoL scores significantly improved at 4 ($P<.01$) and 9 ($P<.001$) months postsurgery.

In a cross-sectional study of 102 patients with CD who underwent TSS (mean time since surgery 7.4 years), 94 patients were confirmed to be in biochemical remission and yet only 81 patients self-identified as such.[23] Biochemical remission after TSS was defined by a postoperative serum cortisol less than 5 ug/dL and/or the need for postoperative CRM. The 13 patients who had achieved biochemical remission but self-identified as having persistent disease (discordant group) reported a higher prevalence of anxiety ($P = .01$) and depression ($P = .02$) via the HADS questionnaire when compared with the 81 patients in biochemical remission who also self-identified as such (concordant group). The concordant group had higher CushingQoL scores ($P = .005$) when compared with the discordant group. Moreover, the study found that in the 94 patients with confirmed biochemical remission, the discordant group had a shorter duration of follow-up (4 years) when compared with the concordant group (7.9 years, $P = .036$), suggesting a delay in psychological versus biochemical recovery. Biochemical remission after TSS was associated with higher CushingQoL scores ($\beta = 14.445$, $P = .015$) and lower depression scores ($\beta = 3.327$, $P = .001$) when compared with remission by alternative therapies (including radiation therapy (RT), adrenalectomy and medical therapy). Interestingly, lower CushingQoL scores were associated with higher BMI ($B = -1.040$, $P = .002$) and longer self-assessed recovery times ($\beta = -0.126$, $P = .024$). These results in conjunction with other studies indicate that CS patients' self-identified remission status is a factor in overall HRQoL scores.[23,37] Patients in biochemical remission who also perceive themselves as such have greater HRQoL scores compared with those in biochemical remission who do not. These findings may help predict which patients are at higher risk for long-term psychopathology.[23]

Several studies have investigated predictive factors for HRQoL after surgery in patients with CD. A prospective study of 17 patients with CD found that while 76.5% had impaired HRQoL preoperatively when compared with the general population, 35.3% of these patients still had impaired HRQoL postoperatively, as assessed by Tuebingen CD-25.[38,39] The study found statistically significant improvements in some domains after surgery, including decreased sexual activity (58.8% improved to 35.3%), bodily restrictions (70.6% improved to 58.8%), disturbed eating behavior (58.8% improved to 5.9%), and cognitive impairment (82.4% improved to 52.9%), but did not find improvement in depressive symptoms.[38] Further analysis found that the number of postoperative comorbidities ($R^2 = 0.441$, $P <.01$) and the decline in morning cortisol level after surgery ($P<.01$) were the strongest predictors of postoperative HRQoL. Patients with more than 2 comorbidities scored lower on the Tuebingen CD-25 than did patients with 2 or less comorbidities. Moreover, greater decreases in morning cortisol levels after surgery resulted in better postoperative HRQoL. On the other hand, younger age was predictive of improved postoperative HRQoL, with improvement in eating behavior being the domain that correlated the best with improvement in younger patients.[38] There was no correlation between time as surgery with postoperative HRQoL in this study or in other studies that included both patients with CS and CD.[28,36,38]

Some studies show gender differences with respect to HRQoL after surgery. In a cohort of 102 patients with CD treated with TSS confirmed to be in biochemical remission, male sex predicted less anxiety using the HADS questionnaire ($\beta = -1.965$, $P = .031$).[23] Another cross-sectional study of 176 patients with CD after TSS found that women were more affected than men in regard to eating behavior and cognition on the Tuebingen CD-25.[40] However, both of these studies included more women than men.[23,40]

A cross-sectional study of 269 patients with CS showed that diagnostic delay (assessed via patient survey as the number of symptomatic years without a diagnosis; median time 5 years) negatively correlated with CushingQoL scores ($r = -0.21$, $P<.001$).[41] Depression was also predictive for outcomes. For example, in a study by Sonino and colleagues that followed 162 patients with CD for at least 2 years after surgery, major depression was present beforehand in 70.8% of patients who had unsuccessful surgeries compared with 43% of patients who had successful surgeries (defined by biochemical remission without the need for further therapies).[42] The same study also found that preoperative major depression resulted in a higher likelihood of relapse for the first 7 years of follow-up, with relapse defined as recurrence of clinical and biochemical characteristics of CS more than 6 months after cure. In another study by Lambert and colleagues that included 346 patients with CD, 22% reported depression at diagnosis.[43] The study further classified these patients postoperatively into 3 subgroups: immediate surgical remission (postoperative hypocortisolemia), late remission (eucortisolemia or hypocortisolemia achieved only after further treatments such as RT or adrenalectomy) and persistent disease. Depression at presentation was shown to increase the risk of death among patients who achieved immediate and late remission (hazard ratio (HR): 6.77, $P = .007$ for the immediate remission subgroup and HR: 4.99, $P = .015$ for the overall remission group). Moreover, preoperative depression was found to predict cardiovascular events among the entire cohort (HR: 2.32, $P = .036$).[43] These studies suggest that depression may be a marker for disease severity and a prognostic indicator for future outcomes.[42,43]

RADIOTHERAPY TREATMENT AND HEALTH-RELATED QUALITY OF LIFE IN CUSHING'S DISEASE

RT can be considered for patients with CD who fail to achieve remission after surgery, patients with aggressive tumors, and when repeat surgery is not feasible or advised. The most common adverse effect of RT is hypopituitarism; 13% to 56% of patients developed pituitary deficits with conventional RT.[44] The development of hypopituitarism and delay in effect, with the need for ongoing cortisol-lowering pharmacotherapy in the interim, are factors that affect HRQoL. While the presence of hypopituitarism after treatment (TSS or RT) affects HRQoL in patients with CD, including worse scores for anxiety and depression via HADS,[36] there are little data on the effects on HRQoL due to hypopituitarism secondary to RT treatment specifically. Given the limited studies, data are mixed regarding postoperative RT and HRQoL in patients with CD.[36,45,46]

In a cross-sectional study of 102 patients with treated CD, Carluccio and colleagues found that remission from TSS was associated with improved HRQoL compared with remission via RT and bilateral adrenalectomy in CD.[23] The authors postulated that this was likely because the latter treatments are recommended for persistent disease, and, in the case of RT, can take several months to years to take effect. Thus, these patients have prolonged exposure to elevated cortisol levels.[23]

However, another study found that 11 patients with CD with a mean of 13.4 years of biochemical remission after RT did not report worse HRQoL scores as measured by SF-36, when compared with an age-adjusted cohort of patients with non-CD.[36] The same was also shown by Webb and colleagues in which prior pituitary RT in 24 patients with CD versus 81 nonirradiated patients with CD did not identify differences in the CushingQoL score.[28]

In a recent study analyzing 69 patients with pituitary adenomas who received RT, PROs were reported for 20 patients.[47] The investigators created a questionnaire regarding current symptoms, imaging, and follow-up treatments. The most common symptoms were fatigue, cognitive disorders, visual decline, dizziness, and vertigo. The study then compared PROs from these 20 patients with the physician-reported outcomes of the same patients according to the CTCAE (common terminology criteria for adverse events). Similar to findings from studies reporting outcomes after surgery,[34] patient and physician outcomes after RT were discordant; patients reported higher incidences of fatigue, vertigo, cognitive disorders, and vision loss than did physicians. It is clear more research is needed to characterize PROs after RT in patients with CS, given the few studies available directly evaluating these measures in this population.

HEALTH-RELATED QUALITY OF LIFE AND MEDICAL TREATMENT OF CUSHING'S SYNDROME

Several recent clinical trials have investigated new medical therapies for CS.[48] CS Medications can be classified as pituitary directed (pasireotide and cabergoline), steroidogenesis inhibitors (ketoconazole, levoketoconazole, metyrapone, osilodrosat, etomidate, and mitotane), and glucocorticoid receptor antagonists (mifepristone).[49] The following section focuses on clinical trials that have explored the effects of medical therapy on HRQoL.

Pasireotide

A phase 3 randomized, multi-center clinical trial including 162 patients with CD determined that the somatostatin analog pasireotide normalized mUFC in 13% of patients treated with 600 μg twice daily and 25% of patients treated with 900 μg twice daily.[14] Subsequent analysis examined the effect of pasireotide on HRQoL and the relationship between HRQoL and 24-hour UFC.[15] Overall, greater than 60% of patients with controlled mUFC, and more than 70% of patients with controlled or partially controlled mUFC ($\geq$50% reduction from baseline) met the CushingQoL MID for improvement at month 12, whereas only one-third of those in the uncontrolled group (mUFC $>$ ULN and $<$50% reduction from baseline) met this threshold. The study showed a statistically significant correlation between changes in CushingQoL score and mUFC at month 12 ($r = -0.40$), but not at month 6, suggesting that HRQoL improved with improved disease control.

A significant relationship was also observed between BDI-II and CushingQoL scores in this cohort. The strongest correlation observed was between baseline BDI-II total score and CushingQoL total score (r = −0.70, $P<.001$). Higher BDI-II scores (indicating more severe depression) were associated with lower CushingQoL scores (reflecting worse HRQoL). Changes in CushingQoL score also correlated with changes in BDI-II at 6 (r = −0.54, $P<.01$) and 12 months (r = −0.59, $P<.01$). Additionally, significant correlations ($P<.01$) were found between changes in CushingQoL score and changes in BMI at 6 (r = −0.39) and 12 months (r = −0.31), as well as weight at 6 (r = −0.41) and 12 months (−0.59).

The above findings were consistent in a real-world, clinical-practice study which showed an effective reduction in mUFC with subcutaneous pasireotide, in addition to improved clinical signs, symptoms, and HRQoL.[50] Another study similarly found improvement in clinical signs and CushingQoL score over 12 months with long-acting pasireotide treatment.[51]

Levoketoconazole

A phase 3, multicenter, open-label, single-arm study demonstrated that treatment with levoketoconazole normalized mUFC in 30% of patients with CS (N = 94, 85% with CD).[52] Secondary endpoints included changes in signs and symptoms, HRQoL, and depression from baseline through month 6.[53]

Significant improvements were seen in mean total scores for acne ($P = .0063$), hirsutism ($P = .0008$), and peripheral edema ($P = .0295$) from baseline to month 6. There was no statistically significant change in the total score for the 7 items evaluated for Cushingoid appearance (moon facies, facial plethora, striae, bruising, supraclavicular fat, irregular menstruation, and dysmenorrhea (in women)). Additionally, there was no significant linear relationship between changes in mUFC and changes in acne, hirsutism, or peripheral edema.

CushingQoL mean scores improved from baseline to month 3 and month 6 of the maintenance phase, with a mean change of 6.9 ($P = .0018$) at months 3 and 10.6 ($P<.0001$) at month 6. Of note, the MID was met or exceeded by 40% of patients at month 3% and 47.1% of patient at month 6. BDI-II mean scores also improved with treatment, with statistically significant improvements seen at month 6 ($P = .0043$). There was no significant relationship between changes in mUFC from baseline to 6 months and changes in CushingQoL or BDI-II score over the same time period.

Mifepristone

In a 24-week, multicenter, open-label trial, clinical outcomes were assessed in 50 endogenous patients with CS treated with the glucocorticoid and progesterone receptor antagonist mifepristone.[54] Study participants were required to have DM, impaired glucose tolerance, or hypertension, with primary endpoints for the study being change in the area under the curve for oral glucose tolerance test from baseline to week 24 in the DM/impaired glucose tolerance cohort and change in diastolic blood pressure from baseline to week 24 in the hypertension cohort. Secondary endpoints included changes in BDI-II score, SF-36, and Trail Making Test A and B (TMT),[55] a neurocognitive processing and executive function assessment.

The primary outcome was met in 60% of the DM cohort, and 38.1% in the hypertension cohort. Overall, median BDI-II scores improved in the modified intention-to-treat group from baseline to week 24 ($P<.001$). TMT scores also showed improvement in cognitive efficiency and executive function (both $P<.01$). Improvement in HRQoL was seen with improved SF-36 mental composite score ($P = .01$) and physical composite score ($P = .02$).

Osilodrostat

Osilodrostat inhibits 11beta-hydroxylase, the enzyme that catalyzes the final step in cortisol synthesis in the adrenal cortex. A prospective, multi-center, randomized withdrawal phase III study showed that twice daily osilodrostat was effective in reducing mUFC compared with the placebo group (86% vs 29%, *P*<.0001) in patients with persistent or recurrent CD (N = 137).[56] Secondary endpoints included CS signs and symptoms, CushingQoL, BDI-II, and EuroQoL scores. Although not extensively detailed in this study, CushingQoL and BDI-II scores improved, by 52.4% and 31.8%, respectively, by week 48, and did meet the MID threshold for both of these assessments. Statistical significance was not directly reported on these outcomes.

LONG-TERM OUTCOMES

PROs improve but may not completely normalize after successful treatment of CS, even after long-term follow-up. Studies have shown that patients with CS who have achieved surgical remission still have poorer HRQoL than healthy controls as measured by various health-related questionnaires.[17,36,46,57–60] This may be due to the persistent effects of prior excess cortisol exposure,[61] or differences in the definitions of CS remission resulting in heterogeneity in remitted cohorts. Some of the most common symptoms that may persist after long-term (mean of 3–13 years) surgical remission in patients with CS include fatigue, trouble sleeping, forgetfulness, weight gain, muscle weakness, anxiety, and depression.[46] Wagenmakers and colleagues assessed HRQoL in 123 patients with pituitary and adrenal CS who had achieved remission for a mean of 13.3 ± 10.4 years, using 7 validated questionnaires including the CushingQoL, HADS, and RAND-36.[59] They found that HRQoL was significantly worse in almost all aspects as compared with controls with the exception of health change and emotional role limitation on the RAND-36, regardless of etiology, presence of hypopituitarism, and treatment strategies including TSS, adrenalectomy, RT or a combination of these. Additionally, as shown elsewhere[36] remission duration did not affect HRQoL on most dimensions, with the exception of depression on HADS, and concentration on 3 assessments: Checklist Individual Strength Questionnaire (CIS), Cognitive Failures Questionnaire, and CushingQoL. Patients with a shorter remission duration scored lower on these dimensions, suggesting that difficulty coping with the diagnosis and sequelae may improve over time.[59]

There have been conflicting results on the effect of hypopituitarism on long-term HRQoL in patients with CS. In a study of 595 patients with CS who completed the CushingQoL and/or EQ-5D questionnaire at baseline and at long-term follow-up, hypopituitarism was not associated with worse HRQoL.[45] Additional studies corroborated these findings,[23,28,62,63] whereas others showed that hypopituitarism negatively impacts several aspects of HRQoL.[36,64] Wagenmakers and colleagues found that patients with CS in remission without hypopituitarism or hormonal deficiencies caused by bilateral adrenalectomy scored significantly better than those without deficiencies on fatigue and motivation, as assessed by CIS and CushingQoL, and energy as assessed by the Nottingham Health Profile (NHP). Patients without hormonal deficiencies also did not have worse HRQoL than the control group on approximately 50% of the items measured, although HRQoL was worse in the other 50% of quality measures. Nevertheless, after multivariate regression analysis, there were persistent impairments in HRQoL in patients with CS in long-term remission regardless of hypopituitarism status.[59] The authors suggest that any further impact of hormone deficiencies on HRQoL may be masked by the overwhelming effect of prior glucocorticoid excess.[45]

The role of bilateral adrenalectomy in long-term HRQoL in patients with CS has also not been clarified, but may be associated with additional symptom burden compared with other treatments. One study compared long-term HRQoL in 17 patients with CD who underwent bilateral adrenalectomy to 17 patients with CD in remission after TSS, medical therapy, or RT. Patients treated with bilateral adrenalectomy scored significantly worse on most aspects of all 3 questionnaires analyzed: SF-36, CushingQoL, and BDI.[65] An earlier study showed lower SF-36 scores in patients who underwent successful bilateral adrenalectomy compared with the general population.[66]

There are contradictory data on whether persistent comorbidities such as hypertension, diabetes, and osteoporosis significantly impact HRQoL in remitted patients, although depression at baseline has consistently predicted lower HRQoL.[13,23,45] One study[23] found that elevated BMI had the strongest negative impact on HRQoL compared with other predictors, as measured by CushingQoL. Another small study of 17 patients with CD in remission found that having 2 postoperative comorbidities such as hypertension, hyperlipidemia, central obesity, or persistent diabetes, was a predictor of poorer HRQoL as measured by the Tuebingen CD-25.[38] Some suggest that using objective data such as blood pressure measurements, Hemoglobin A1c, and lipid profiles to assess comorbidities, rather than self-reported data, may lead to more accurate evaluations of the relationships between comorbidities and HRQoL.[23]

Smaller studies on potential HRQoL differences among pituitary versus adrenal CS have produced discordant results.[28,30,59,63] Valassi and colleagues performed the largest review to date on this topic.[45] They found that at long-term follow-up, pituitary CS had worse HRQoL when compared with patients with adrenal CS. However, there was no difference between these 2 groups when only patients in remission were analyzed. The authors concluded that remission was the most important predictor of a favorable outcome for the CushingQoL, which strongly indicates that hypercortisolism is the main determinant for long-term HRQoL impairment in CS.

SUMMARY AND FUTURE DIRECTIONS

Patients with active CS experience a wide range of signs and symptoms, and notably report impaired HRQoL when compared with patients who have achieved remission and normative controls. Impaired HRQoL and ongoing depression and anxiety may persist even after surgical remission,[36,46,57–60] possibly related to ongoing comorbidities or persistent effects of prior glucocorticoid exposure. For patients treated with RT, PROs may be affected by hypopituitarism and delay in achieving remission. Recent and ongoing advances in medical therapies for CS allow for more treatment options for patients which could improve long-term PROs.

Educating patients on expectations during and after treatment may help them prepare for the possibility of reduced HRQoL despite biochemical control. Periodic, lifelong screening and care of persistent comorbidities posttreatment are essential. A multidisciplinary approach consisting of skilled physicians, support groups, family members, and educational tools such as brochures or seminars should be used to manage patients' long term.[67] Ongoing educational programs that assess comorbidities and provide specific physical activity and dietary guidelines have been shown to improve CushingQoL scores, reduce pain, increase physical activity, and promote a healthier lifestyle.[68] Thus, group programs such as these have shown encouraging results, but there is still a need for development.[17,69]

Further research is needed to assess critical PROs in patients receiving long-term medical treatment. This will help guide the direction of ongoing and future medical therapy development with the critical focus of developing therapies that address the symptom burden that patients with CS may experience despite successful treatment.

CLINICS CARE POINTS

- Health-related quality of life can be measured in this population before and after treatment using the CushingQoL and Tuebingen CD-25, 2 disease-specific questionnaires.
- In patients with active Cushing's syndrome, it is important to screen for major depression, as this comorbidity has been shown to directly impact health-related quality of life.
- Clinicians should foster open communication and provide patients with objective information on expected symptoms during and after treatment.
- Perform periodic, life-long evaluations in patients with CS to ensure comorbidities are properly managed after treatment.
- When managing patients in long-term biochemical remission, educate them on the possibility of persistent symptoms and reduced health-related quality of life; ensure adequate support in the form of educational resources and group programs.

DISCLOSURE

E.B. Geer reports serving as an investigator for research grants to MSKCC from Recordati, Strongbridge/Xeris, and Corcept; and serving as an occasional consultant to Xeris. Remaining authors have nothing to disclose.

REFERENCES

1. Hakami OA, Ahmed S, Karavitaki N. Epidemiology and mortality of Cushing's syndrome. Best Pract Res Clin Endocrinol Metab 2021;35(1):101521.
2. Knoble N, Nayroles G, Cheng C, et al. Illustration of patient-reported outcome challenges and solutions in rare diseases: A systematic review in Cushing's syndrome. Orphanet J Rare Dis 2018;13(1):1–10.
3. Weldring T, Smith SMS. Article Commentary: Patient-Reported Outcomes (PROs) and Patient-Reported Outcome Measures (PROMs). Health Serv Insights 2013; 6:61–8.
4. Nieman LK. Cushing's syndrome: Update on signs, symptoms and biochemical screening. Eur J Endocrinol 2015;173(4):M33–8.
5. Santos A, Resmini E, Pascual JC, et al. Psychiatric Symptoms in Patients with Cushing's Syndrome: Prevalence, Diagnosis and Management. Drugs 2017; 77(8):829–42.
6. Valassi E, Santos A, Yaneva M, et al. The European Registry on Cushing's syndrome: 2-Year experience. Baseline demographic and clinical characteristics. Eur J Endocrinol 2011;165(3):383–92.
7. Webb SM, Santos A, Aulinas A, et al. Patient-Centered Outcomes with Pituitary and Parasellar Disease. Neuroendocrinology 2020;110(9–10):882–8.
8. Na S, Fernandes MA, Ioachimescu AG, et al. Neuropsychological and Emotional Functioning in Patients with Cushing's Syndrome. Behav Neurol 2020;2020. https://doi.org/10.1155/2020/4064370.

9. Starkman MN, Schteingart DE, Schork MA. Depressed mood and other psychiatric manifestations of Cushing's syndrome: relationship to hormone levels. Psychosom Med 1981;43(1):3–18.
10. Loosen PT, Chambliss B, DeBold CR, et al. Psychiatric phenomenology in Cushing's disease. Pharmacopsychiatry 1992;25(4):192–8.
11. Kelly WF. Psychiatric aspects of Cushing's syndrome. QJM 1996;89(7):543–52.
12. Santos A, Resmini E, Crespo I, et al. Small cerebellar cortex volume in patients with active Cushing's syndrome. Eur J Endocrinol 2014;171(4):461–9.
13. Badia X, Valassi E, Roset M, et al. Disease-specific quality of life evaluation and its determinants in Cushing's syndrome: What have we learnt? Pituitary 2014; 17(2):187–95.
14. Colao A, Petersenn S, Newell-Price J, et al. A 12-Month Phase 3 Study of Pasireotide in Cushing's Disease. N Engl J Med 2012;366(10):914–24.
15. Webb SM, Ware JE, Forsythe A, et al. Treatment effectiveness of pasireotide on health-related quality of life in patients with Cushing's disease. Eur J Endocrinol 2014;171(1):89–98.
16. Huguet I, Ntali G, Grossman A, et al. Cushing's disease - Quality of life, recurrence and long-term morbidity. Eur Endocrinol 2015;11(1):34–8.
17. Santos A, Resmini E, Martinez Momblan MA, et al. Quality of Life in Patients With Cushing's Disease. Front Endocrinol (Lausanne) 2019;10:862.
18. Busija L, Pausenberger E, Haines TP, et al. Adult measures of general health and health-related quality of life: Medical Outcomes Study Short Form 36-Item (SF-36) and Short Form 12-Item (SF-12) Health Surveys, Nottingham Health Profile (NHP), Sickness Impact Profile (SIP), Medical Outcomes Study Short Form 6D (SF-6D), Health Utilities Index Mark 3 (HUI3), Quality of Well-Being Scale (QWB), and Assessment of Quality of Life (AQoL). Arthritis Care Res (Hoboken) 2011; 63(Suppl 11):S383–412.
19. Abbasi-Ghahramanloo A, Soltani-Kermanshahi M, Mansori K, et al. Comparison of SF-36 and WHOQoL-BREF in Measuring Quality of Life in Patients with Type 2 Diabetes. Int J Gen Med 2020;13:497–506.
20. Webb SM, Crespo I, Santos A, et al. Quality of life tools for the management of pituitary disease. Eur J Endocrinol 2017;177(1):R13–26.
21. Milian M, Teufel P, Honegger J, et al. The development of the Tuebingen Cushing's disease quality of life inventory (Tuebingen CD-25). Part I: Construction and psychometric properties. Clin Endocrinol 2012;76(6):851–60.
22. Julian LJ. Measures of anxiety: State-Trait Anxiety Inventory (STAI), Beck Anxiety Inventory (BAI), and Hospital Anxiety and Depression Scale-Anxiety (HADS-A). Arthritis Care Res (Hoboken) 2011;63:S467–72. Suppl 11(0 11).
23. Carluccio A, Sundaram NK, Chablani S, et al. Predictors of quality of life in 102 patients with treated Cushing's disease. Clin Endocrinol (Oxf) 2015;82(3):404–11.
24. Button KS, Kounali D, Thomas L, et al. Minimal clinically important difference on the Beck Depression Inventory–II according to the patient's perspective. Psychol Med 2015;45(15):3269–79.
25. Hewlett S, Dures E, Almeida C. Measures of fatigue: Bristol Rheumatoid Arthritis Fatigue Multi-Dimensional Questionnaire (BRAF MDQ), Bristol Rheumatoid Arthritis Fatigue Numerical Rating Scales (BRAF NRS) for severity, effect, and coping, Chalder Fatigue Questionnaire (CFQ), Checklist Individual Strength (CIS20R and CIS8R), Fatigue Severity Scale (FSS), Functional Assessment Chronic Illness Therapy (Fatigue) (FACIT-F), Multi-Dimensional Assessment of Fatigue (MAF), Multi-Dimensional Fatigue Inventory (MFI), Pediatric Quality Of Life (PedsQL) Multi-Dimensional Fatigue Scale, Profile of Fatigue (ProF), Short Form

36 Vitality Subscale (SF-36 VT), and Visual Analog Scales (VAS). Arthritis Care Res (Hoboken) 2011;63(Suppl 11):S263–86.
26. Keskin FE, Özkaya HM, Ortaç M, et al. Sexual function in women with cushing's syndrome: A controlled study. Turkish J Urol 2018;44(4):287–93.
27. Omachi TA. Measures of sleep in rheumatologic diseases: Epworth Sleepiness Scale (ESS), Functional Outcome of Sleep Questionnaire (FOSQ), Insomnia Severity Index (ISI), and Pittsburgh Sleep Quality Index (PSQI). Arthritis Care Res (Hoboken) 2011;63:S287–96. Suppl 11(0 11).
28. Webb SM, Badia X, Barahona MJ, et al. Evaluation of health-related quality of life in patients with Cushing's syndrome with a new questionnaire. Eur J Endocrinol 2008;158(5):623–30.
29. Nelson LM, Forsythe A, McLeod L, et al. Psychometric evaluation of the Cushing's Quality-of-Life questionnaire. The patient 2013;6(2):113–24.
30. Webb SM, Crespo I, Santos A, et al. MANAGEMENT OF ENDOCRINE DISEASE: Quality of life tools for the management of pituitary disease. Eur J Endocrinol 2017;177(1):R13–26.
31. Johnston BC, Ebrahim S, Carrasco-Labra A, et al. Minimally important difference estimates and methods: A protocol. BMJ Open 2015;5(10):1–7.
32. Santos A, Resmini E, Martinez-Momblan MA, et al. Psychometric performance of the CushingQoL questionnaire in conditions of real clinical practice. Eur J Endocrinol 2012;167(3):337–42.
33. Milian M, Teufel P, Honegger J, et al. The development of the Tuebingen Cushing's disease quality of life inventory (Tuebingen CD-25). Part II: Normative data from 1784 healthy people. Clin Endocrinol 2012;76(6):861–7.
34. Acree R, Miller CM, Abel BS, et al. Patient and Provider Perspectives on Postsurgical Recovery of Cushing Syndrome. J Endocr Soc 2021;5(8):bvab109.
35. Webb SM, Santos A, Resmini E, et al. Quality of Life in Cushing's disease: A long term issue? Ann Endocrinol (Paris) 2018;79(3):132–7.
36. van Aken MO, Pereira AM, Biermasz NR, et al. Quality of life in patients after long-term biochemical cure of Cushing's disease. J Clin Endocrinol Metab 2005;90(6): 3279–86.
37. Tiemensma J, Kaptein AA, Pereira AM, et al. Negative illness perceptions are associated with impaired quality of life in patients after long-term remission of Cushing's syndrome. Eur J Endocrinol 2011;165(4):527–35.
38. Milian M, Honegger J, Teufel P, et al. Tuebingen CD-25 Is a Sensitive Tool to Investigate Health-Related Quality of Life in Cushing's Disease Patients in the Course of the Disease. Neuroendocrinology 2013;98(3):188–99.
39. Milian M, Kreitschmann-Andermahr I, Siegel S, et al. Validation of the Tuebingen CD-25 Inventory as a Measure of Postoperative Health-Related Quality of Life in Patients Treated for Cushing's Disease. Neuroendocrinology 2015;102(1–2):60–7.
40. Siegel S, Milian M, Kleist B, et al. Coping strategies have a strong impact on quality of life, depression, and embitterment in patients with Cushing's disease. Pituitary 2016;19(6):590–600.
41. Papoian V, Biller BMK, Webb S, et al. Patients' Perception On Clinical Outcome And Quality Of Life After A Diagnosis Of Cushing Syndrome. Endocr Pract 2015;22. https://doi.org/10.4158/EP15855.OR.
42. Sonino N, Zielezny M, Fava GA, et al. Risk factors and long-term outcome in pituitary-dependent Cushing's disease. J Clin Endocrinol Metab 1996;81(7): 2647–52.

43. Lambert JK, Goldberg L, Fayngold S, et al. Predictors of mortality and long-term outcomes in treated Cushing's disease: a study of 346 patients. J Clin Endocrinol Metab 2013;98(3):1022–30.
44. Castinetti F, Brue T, Ragnarsson O. Radiotherapy as a tool for the treatment of Cushing's disease. Eur J Endocrinol 2019;180(5):D9–18.
45. Valassi E, Feelders R, Maiter D, et al. Worse Health-Related Quality of Life at long-term follow-up in patients with Cushing's disease than patients with cortisol producing adenoma. Data from the ERCUSYN. Clin Endocrinol (Oxf) 2018;88(6): 787–98.
46. Lindsay JR, Nansel T, Baid S, et al. Long-term impaired quality of life in Cushing's syndrome despite initial improvement after surgical remission. J Clin Endocrinol Metab 2006;91(2):447–53.
47. Kessel KA, Diehl CD, Oechsner M, et al. Patient-Reported Outcome (PRO) as an Addition to Long-Term Results after High-Precision Stereotactic Radiotherapy in Patients with Secreting and Non-Secreting Pituitary Adenomas: A Retrospective Cohort Study up to 17-Years Follow-Up. Cancers (Basel) 2019;11(12). https://doi.org/10.3390/cancers11121884.
48. Broersen LHA, Jha M, Biermasz NR, et al. Effectiveness of medical treatment for Cushing's syndrome: a systematic review and meta-analysis. Pituitary 2018; 21(6):631–41.
49. Pivonello R, Ferrigno R, De Martino MC, et al. Medical Treatment of Cushing's Disease: An Overview of the Current and Recent Clinical Trials. Front Endocrinol 2020;11. https://doi.org/10.3389/fendo.2020.00648.
50. Fleseriu M, Iweha C, Salgado L, et al. Safety and efficacy of subcutaneous pasireotide in patients with Cushing's disease: Results from an open-label, multicenter, single-arm, multinational, expanded-access study. Front Endocrinol 2019;10. https://doi.org/10.3389/fendo.2019.00436.
51. Lacroix A, Bronstein MD, Schopohl J, et al. Long-acting pasireotide improves clinical signs and quality of life in Cushing's disease: results from a phase III study. J Endocrinol Invest 2020;43(11):1613–22.
52. Fleseriu M, Pivonello R, Elenkova A, et al. Efficacy and safety of levoketoconazole in the treatment of endogenous Cushing's syndrome (SONICS): a phase 3, multicentre, open-label, single-arm trial. Lancet Diabetes Endocrinol 2019;7(11): 855–65.
53. Geer EB, Salvatori R, Elenkova A, et al. Levoketoconazole improves clinical signs and symptoms and patient-reported outcomes in patients with Cushing's syndrome. Pituitary 2021;24(1):104–15.
54. Fleseriu M, Biller BMK, Findling JW, et al. Mifepristone, a glucocorticoid receptor antagonist, produces clinical and metabolic benefits in patients with Cushing's syndrome. J Clin Endocrinol Metab 2012;97(6):2039–49.
55. Papakokkinou E, Johansson B, Berglund P, et al. Mental Fatigue and Executive Dysfunction in Patients with Cushing's Syndrome in Remission. Behav Neurol 2015;2015. https://doi.org/10.1155/2015/173653.
56. Pivonello R, Fleseriu M, Newell-Price J, et al. Efficacy and safety of osilodrostat in patients with Cushing's disease (LINC 3): a multicentre phase III study with a double-blind, randomised withdrawal phase. Lancet Diabetes Endocrinol 2020; 8(9):748–61.
57. Vermalle M, Alessandrini M, Graillon T, et al. Lack of functional remission in Cushing's syndrome. Endocrine 2018;61(3):518–25.

58. Nader S, Burkhardt T, Vettorazzi E, et al. Health-related Quality of Life in Patients After Treatment of Cushing's Disease. Exp Clin Endocrinol Diabetes 2016;124(3): 187–91.
59. Wagenmakers MA, Netea-Maier RT, Prins JB, et al. Impaired quality of life in patients in long-term remission of Cushing's syndrome of both adrenal and pituitary origin: a remaining effect of long-standing hypercortisolism? Eur J Endocrinol 2012;167(5):687–95.
60. Forget H, Lacroix A, Cohen H. Persistent cognitive impairment following surgical treatment of Cushing's syndrome. Psychoneuroendocrinology 2002;27(3): 367–83.
61. Lacroix A, Feelders RA, Stratakis CA, et al. Cushing's syndrome. Lancet 2015; 386(9996):913–27.
62. Raappana A, Pirilä T, Ebeling T, et al. Long-term health-related quality of life of surgically treated pituitary adenoma patients: a descriptive study. ISRN Endocrinol 2012;2012:675310.
63. Lindholm J, Juul S, Jørgensen JO, et al. Incidence and late prognosis of cushing's syndrome: a population-based study. J Clin Endocrinol Metab 2001;86(1): 117–23.
64. van der Klaauw AA, Kars M, Biermasz NR, et al. Disease-specific impairments in quality of life during long-term follow-up of patients with different pituitary adenomas. Clin Endocrinol (Oxf) 2008;69(5):775–84.
65. Sarkis P, Rabilloud M, Lifante JC, et al. Bilateral adrenalectomy in Cushing's disease: Altered long-term quality of life compared to other treatment options. Ann Endocrinol (Paris) 2019;80(1):32–7.
66. Hawn MT, Cook D, Deveney C, et al. Quality of life after laparoscopic bilateral adrenalectomy for Cushing's disease. Surgery 2002;132(6):1064–8 [discussion: 1068–9].
67. Kreitschmann-Andermahr I, Siegel S, Gammel C, et al. Support Needs of Patients with Cushing's Disease and Cushing's Syndrome: Results of a Survey Conducted in Germany and the USA. Int J Endocrinol 2018;2018:9014768.
68. Martínez-Momblán MA, Gómez C, Santos A, et al. A specific nursing educational program in patients with Cushing's syndrome. Endocrine 2016;53(1):199–209.
69. Bride MM, Crespo I, Webb SM, et al. Quality of life in Cushing's syndrome. Best Pract Res Clin Endocrinol Metab 2021;35(1):101505.

Evaluating the Impact of Acromegaly on Quality of Life

Eva C. Coopmans, MD, PhD[a,b,*], Cornelie D. Andela, MD, PhD[a,b,c], Kim M.J.A. Claessen, MD, PhD[a,b], Nienke R. Biermasz, MD, PhD[a,b,*]

KEYWORDS

- Acromegaly • Somatotropinoma • Comorbidities • Quality of life
- Patient-reported outcomes

KEY POINTS

- Although metabolic alterations, hypertension, and the early stages of cardiomyopathy may be reversible after cure or disease control, many other complications such as musculoskeletal disorders can persist even when the disease is controlled. Consequently, the clinical burden due to acromegaly-associated comorbidities may adversely affect the quality of life (QoL).
- Patient-reported outcome measures (PROMs) are pivotal in the evaluation of disease activity. PROMs have added value in guiding treatment decisions, in particular when growth hormone (GH) and insulin-like growth factor I (IGF-1) levels are discrepant, when patients are only partial responders to treatment, or in patients with discrepant results between PROMs and conventional biochemical outcomes.
- A patient-centered approach should be considered in treatment decisions, integrating conventional biochemical outcomes, tumor control, comorbidities, treatment complications, and PROMs, including QoL measures.

INTRODUCTION

Excess levels of circulating GH and IGF-1 in acromegaly have deleterious effects on a wide range of physiologic processes and tissues. GH levels directly reflect somatotroph tumor secretory activity, and IGF-1 levels reflect peripheral disease activity. Unfortunately, there is often a delay in treatment, as it can take several years of symptoms for a patient to be diagnosed with acromegaly.[1] During this delay, irreversible acromegaly-associated comorbidities may develop, including malignant

[a] Department of Medicine, Division of Endocrinology, Leiden University Medical Center, P.O. Box 9600, 2300 RC Leiden, the Netherlands; [b] Center for Endocrine Tumors Leiden (CETL), Center for Pituitary Care, Leiden University Medical Center, Albinusdreef 2, 2333 ZB Leiden, the Netherlands; [c] Basalt Rehabilitation Center, Vrederustlaan 180, 2543 SW Den Haag, the Netherlands
* Corresponding authors. Department of Medicine, Division of Endocrinology, Leiden University Medical Center, P.O. Box 9600, 2300 RC Leiden, the Netherlands.
E-mail addresses: e.c.coopmans@lumc.nl (E.C.C.); n.r.biermasz@lumc.nl (N.R.B.)

Endocrinol Metab Clin N Am 51 (2022) 709–725
https://doi.org/10.1016/j.ecl.2022.04.004 endo.theclinics.com
0889-8529/22/

neoplasm and cancer, cardiovascular disorders, type 2 diabetes mellitus, hypopituitarism, arthropathy, vertebral fractures, and psychological morbidity, all of which may affect mortality risk and/or well-being.[2–8]

Recent advances in acromegaly disease control, as well as improved management of comorbidities, have led to lower mortality rates, approaching those of the general population.[9,10] This is usually achieved by multimodality treatment (eg, a combination of surgery, chronic medical treatment, and radiotherapy). In the last two decades, however, it has become apparent that despite normalization of GH and IGF-1 levels and establishing tumor control, musculoskeletal disorders and several other persistent comorbidities may persist. As a consequence, both active and controlled patients with acromegaly report impairments in quality of life (QoL), and the clinical burden due to acromegaly-associated comorbidities adversely affects QoL.[11–15]

Although effective treatment of acromegaly improves QoL and patients' symptoms, biochemical control does not necessarily correlate with clinical well-being, and QoL impairments often persist despite biochemical control.[11] Therefore, a more patient-centered approach, including conventional biochemical outcomes, comorbidities, treatment complications, and the patient perspective by using patient-reported outcome measures (PROMs), should all be considered in treatment decisions. PROMs can assess any component of a patient's health status that comes directly from the patient, without the interpretation of clinicians or anyone else.[16] PROMs can be used to measure purely somatic or psychological symptoms (eg, pain, weight gain, and depressive thoughts), functional problems (eg, carrying out daily activities such as work and family life), and more complex general health perceptions and QoL. PROMs can be generic assessments of QoL in general (eg, Short Form 36 [SF-36]), domain-specific (ie, Hospital Anxiety and Depression Scale [HADS]), or disease-specific (eg, *Acromegaly Quality of Life questionnaire*[AcroQoL]). When interpreting PROMs, it is important to acknowledge the biopsychosocial character of well-being, as conceptualized by the Wilson and Cleary model.17 To effectively use PROMs for decision-making, it is important to understand the paradigm of how well-being is conceptualized. Following the Wilson and Cleary model, health can be seen as a continuum of increasing biological, psychological, and social complexity, ranging from pure biological factors, symptoms, and functional impairments to general health perceptions, all taking into account the influence of individual and environmental characteristics.

This review aims to discuss the impact of acromegaly on QoL from the clinical perspective as well as from the patient perspective. Furthermore, it aims to evaluate the use of PROMs in acromegaly and how PROMs aid decision-making. The recommendations presented in this review are based on recent clinical evidence on the impact of acromegaly on QoL combined with authors' own clinical experience treating patients with acromegaly.

CLINICAL BURDEN

Patients receiving treatment for acromegaly often experience a significant clinical disease burden. Local mass effects and treatment of the tumor may result in side effects and complications, such as hypopituitarism, visual symptoms, and headache. Furthermore, hormone excess results in specific somatic symptoms (eg, changes in facial appearance, acral growth, fatigue, sweating, and pain) and acromegaly-associated comorbidities (eg, type 2 diabetes mellitus, heart failure, arthropathy, and obstructive sleep apnea [OSA]). The risk of developing one of these characteristic comorbidities is greater relative to that of the general population, with a higher risk for comorbidities observed in patients with biochemically uncontrolled acromegaly.[15,18,19] Although metabolic alterations, hypertension, and early stages of cardiomyopathy may be reversible after early cure or disease control,[20,21] many other complications (eg, musculoskeletal disorders or OSA) may persist or even show progression.[22–25]

Malignant Neoplasm and Cancer

Other neoplasms apart from the pituitary, specifically the prevalence of colon cancer and differentiated thyroid carcinomas, appear to be increased among patients with acromegaly.[26] Cancer is currently the leading cause of mortality,[27–29] although cancer-specific mortality rates in acromegaly are generally similar to those observed in the general population.[27] In addition, increased life expectancy in acromegaly has been associated with more deaths resulting from malignancies that are not typically related to GH or IGF-1 excess. With this in mind, cancer incidence in acromegaly seems to be more related to age than to GH excess, and patients in the modern era may live long enough to reach the age of increased cancer risk.[30] Finally, it should be borne in mind that the increased number of diagnoses of cancer could happen in these patients because they are examined more accurately and more frequently before diagnosis (ie, surveillance bias).

As colonoscopy screening for colonic neoplasia is recommended every 10 years and more frequently in those with persistently elevated IGF-1, having polyps at previous colonoscopies, or in case of a positive family history of colon cancer,[4] it should be kept in mind that screening methods for early cancer detection might lead to significant psychological distress in patients.[31,32]

Cardiovascular Disorders

Cardiovascular events are responsible for increased mortality rates in acromegaly; however, those with well-controlled acromegaly are now closely approximating that of the general population.[27,28]

Subclinical cardiomyopathy with left ventricular hypertrophy is a frequent finding (up to 80% of patients) and is characterized by concentric hypertrophy, progressive systolic deficiency, and diastolic dysfunction. Congestive heart failure may ensue that it is associated with substantial complaints (including loss of energy, reduced exercise tolerance, shortness of breath), functional limitations, and a worse prognosis.

Arterial hypertension is a common finding in up to 60% of acromegaly patients.[8,33] Multifactorial pathogenesis must be assumed in which GH- and IGF-1-mediated sodium and water retention and sympathetic dysfunction seem to play an important role, but hyperinsulinemia and cardiovascular disorder must also be considered.

Endocrine and Metabolic Disorders

Type 2 diabetes mellitus

The most frequent metabolic comorbidities are impaired glucose tolerance and type 2 diabetes mellitus, which are present at diagnosis in up to 50% of patients.[34,35] Owing to GH excess, patients develop insulin resistance, and in the long term, insulin insufficiency with impaired glucose tolerance may occur.[36] Although there are no available studies evaluating the outcome of diabetes complications in acromegaly, microangiopathic complications occur relatively early in the disease course, suggesting a role of GH. As acromegaly patients with diabetes have a higher prevalence of dyslipidemia and hypertension but are also at increased risk of hypertrophic cardiomyopathy with severe diastolic dysfunction, mortality is increased in this subset of patients.[37,38] Previous studies showed that having diabetes mellitus affects QoL adversely in patients with acromegaly.[39,40]

As nearly all patients at diagnosis undergo oral glucose tolerance test, the required information to evaluate the glycemic status is available. Accordingly, if type 2 diabetes is diagnosed, it should be managed for the general population.

Hypopituitarism

Hypopituitarism has been observed in more than 40% of patients with acromegaly, especially among patients treated with conventional radiation therapy. Although hormonal substitution therapy has been extremely successful in improving morbidity and mortality, many patients treated for endocrine insufficiencies still suffer from "vague" complaints and experience impairment in QoL.[41] Glucocorticoid replacement is specifically important to mention, because both under-supplementation and over-supplementation are associated with significant morbidity (including adrenal crisis vs dyslipidemia, cardiovascular risk, and further impairment of bone quality) and mortality.[42] Moreover, it is known from previous studies that glucocorticoid replacement therapy is taxing for patients, with the need for several lifestyle adaptations, concerns about side effects of their medication, fear of adrenal crisis, and often suboptimal care at the emergency department.[43]

The development of GH deficiency following acromegaly treatment is also clearly associated with a compromised QoL.[14,39,44] Hypogonadotropic hypogonadism occurs in more than 50% of patients, either caused by hypopituitarism from tumor mass effect or hyperprolactinemia.[45] On acromegaly treatment, semen quality and androgen levels (total testosterone, sex hormone-binding globulin) do not always fully recover, which has not only substantial consequences for the sexual and reproductive ability but also affects body composition, glucose homeostasis, and energy level. Therefore, regular evaluation of the gonadal axis is needed, and testosterone supplementation should be considered on an individual basis.

Long-term monitoring for the development of hormonal deficit and signs of under-supplementation and over-supplementation is recommended annually, particularly in those who have received radiotherapy, with a clear need for optimization and individualization of supplementation regimens.[19]

Obstructive sleep apnea

Up to 80% of patients suffer from OSA as a result of macroglossia and soft-tissue pharyngeal swelling,[23,35,46–49] but some patients also present with central sleep apnea. Although the soft tissue swelling improves after adequate treatment of GH excess, there is an irreversible remodeling of the upper airways in acromegaly with the persistence of OSA after biochemical cure in most patients. OSA results in headaches, poor sleep quality, daily somnolence, and impaired neurocognitive function in acromegaly patients. Moreover, in observational studies, OSA is related to insulin resistance, hypertension, heart failure, arrhythmias, and cerebrovascular disease.[50] Thereby, OSA has a major negative impact on physical, social, and psychological functioning and predisposes to morbidity and mortality.[51–53]

Owing to the high prevalence of OSA in acromegaly, thorough history taking, questioning of spouse/partner, and potentially use of a PROM (ie, Epworth sleepiness scale [ESS][54]) is necessary. In cases of strong suspicion, polysomnography may be performed, even before transsphenoidal surgery.

Musculoskeletal Disorders

Arthropathy

Arthropathy is one of the most frequent complications of acromegaly, and arthropathy pain is one of the most prominent symptoms negatively affecting QoL.[55] GH and IGF-1 excess induces cartilage hypertrophy and osteophyte formation that contribute to joint space narrowing, with generally degenerative but no inflammatory changes. One of the difficulties in the diagnostics of acromegalic arthropathy is the unexplained mismatch between radiologic changes and clinical symptoms, which is well-known in primary osteoarthritis. The knees and spine are particularly affected, but other functionally important joints such as the hands, hips, and shoulders are often involved too. Our recent prospective studies demonstrated that a large subset of patients show the clinical and radiographic progression of the joint disease over time, even after long-term disease control.[56,57] Although treatment of GH and IGF-1 excess is able to improve symptoms in most patients and is thereby the cornerstone in the management of joint symptoms, good biochemical control of acromegaly alone is insufficient to stabilize this chronic, partially irreversible complication in many patients. In some cases, physiotherapy may be beneficial, and in late-stage disease, individual joints may benefit from replacement surgery, but there is only anecdotal evidence of its effectiveness. There is a clear need for optimization of treatment strategies, and we recommend the development of multidisciplinary care for severe joint disease beyond endocrine care only.

Vertebral fractures

GH and IGF-1 excess in acromegaly leads to high bone turnover, deterioration of the cortical and trabecular bone structure, and increased risk of vertebral fractures. More than 50% of individuals with fractures have multiple or severe vertebral fractures, predisposing patients to have back pain, progressive thoracal kyphosis, sagittal imbalance, and thereby functional impairments. In addition, cardiopulmonary complications have a potentially worse outcome in acromegalic patients with (severe) vertebral fractures/deformities.[58] The presence of vertebral fractures is related to increased pain scores and impairments in QoL in patients with acromegaly.[59,60]

Accordingly, fracture risk is highest in patients with long-standing active acromegaly, especially in patients with hypogonadism. However, vertebral fractures can also occur in a later phase of the disease, with a persistently high prevalence and even progression in patients with disease control.[57,61] In the absence of reliable tools to predict the fracture risk in acromegaly patients, we recommend screening all patients for osteoporosis and vertebral fractures by dual-energy x-ray absorptiometry and plain radiographs, respectively, regardless of disease status. Other risk factors, including hypogonadism, vitamin D deficiency, and glucocorticoid over substitution, should be identified and corrected. Although the literature on the efficacy and safety of bone-modifying drugs in acromegaly is limited,[62,63] patients with low bone mineral density values and progressive vertebral fractures are likely to benefit from antiresorptive drugs, especially early in the disease course when bone turnover is high.

Changes in Physical Appearance

Acromegaly is typically associated with excessive sweating and morphometric changes, including enlarged extremities and facial abnormalities, such as furrowing of the forehead, enlargement of the nose and ears, thickening of the lips, and mandibular prognathism. These features significantly improve after the reversal of GH excess but do not always completely normalize.[64–66] Morphometric changes significantly correlate with poor psychological outcomes in acromegaly patients, and it is extremely important to address this subject during consultation.[40,67] GH-induced vocal changes are also frequently reported during active disease, although mucosal edema and hypertrophy largely resolve during treatment with the improvement of symptoms, voice complaints persist in a subset of patients. This also negatively influences QoL, and consultation with a speech therapist could be beneficial.[68]

Issues in Psychosocial Functioning

Even after optimal medical treatment, acromegaly is associated with an increased prevalence of psychopathology and maladaptive personality traits.[13,69] According to Pertichetti *and colleagues*, 63% of acromegalic patients suffer from psychiatric disorders, mostly attributed to depression, followed by psychosis and anxiety.[70] Impairments in cognitive functioning were absent in some studies,[69] whereas others did observe impairments in cognitive functioning, in particular attention deficits, with the occurrence of alterations in brain volume.[71–73]

A recent quantitative study of our research group examined work disability among patients treated for a pituitary tumor. It was shown that a substantial part of pituitary patients had no paid job (28%). Patients with acromegaly or Cushing's disease were more often without a paid job than patients with prolactinoma or nonfunctioning adenoma. Of the pituitary patients who had a paid job, 41% reported health-related absenteeism in the previous year. Most of that impacted work productivity was of mental or social origin.[74] This is in line with the results of a focus group study where patients treated for a pituitary tumor reported work-related problems because of diminished ability to function, concentration problems, and issues with collaborating with others.[75] Besides the psychosocial burden perceived by patients, their partners/spouses also reported a negative impact of the consequences of the disease on their psychosocial well-being.[76]

Furthermore, patients with acromegaly reported more problems with sexual functioning compared with healthy controls, including inability to achieve orgasm and decreased libido. In accordance with the multifactorial nature of sexual functioning, issues in sexual functioning were related to higher IGF-I levels, more depressive symptoms, and older age.[75,77] In focus group conversations with patients with acromegaly, patients attributed their decreased libido to the disease as well as to aging, a negative self-image, shame, physical pain, and as a side effect of their medical therapy.[75]

In the examination of how patients perceive their illness, it was shown that patients with acromegaly report affected illness perceptions,[69] with acromegalic patients receiving medical treatment tending to perceive a more chronic timeline of their disease compared with patients in remission without medical treatment.[78] In patients using medication for acromegaly, negative beliefs about their medication were related to more negative illness perceptions and more impairments in acromegaly-specific QoL (ie, AcroQoL).[78] Moreover, patients reported less effective coping strategies.[79] Clinicians should be aware of these persistent psychosocial issues and potential impairments in cognitive functioning that can be supported by the use of PROMs.

PATIENT-REPORTED OUTCOME MEASURES

A substantial number of clinical trials among patients with acromegaly use PROMs alongside biochemical outcomes.[16] PROMs are now contemplated by health administrators and regulating agencies when considering health-related decisions, such as authorizing reimbursement of new drugs.[4,80] However, no clear criteria nor consensus exists for the use of PROMs in trials of patients with acromegaly. In addition, comparability between trials is limited due to a great variety of validated and unvalidated generic and disease-specific PROMs that are currently being used. Recently, in a large meta-analysis of 53 intervention and cohort studies, the authors showed that of the 14 PROMs that were used in acromegaly patients, only one, the AcroQoL, has been validated in patients with acromegaly.[81]

Generic-specific, domain-specific, and acromegaly-specific QoL measures can help identify specific factors for follow-up. The following is a list of the most commonly used PROMs in acromegaly:

Disease-Specific/Acromegaly-Specific Patient-Reported Outcome Measures

- *AcroQoL Questionnaire:* A disease-specific, self-rating questionnaire that comprises 22 items, with each having five possible answers scoring 1 to 5. The questions are divided into two main categories: physical (8 items) and psychological function (14 items, subdivided into appearance and personal relationships). The score of 110 (100%) represents optimal QoL.[82]
- *Patient-Assessed Acromegaly Symptom Questionnaire (PASQ)*: A disease-specific, self-rating questionnaire that comprises 6 items, with each having nine possible answers scoring 0 to 8. These questions evaluate symptoms and signs of acromegaly, such as headache, excessive perspiration, osteoarthralgia, fatigue, soft-tissue swelling, and paresthesia. The seventh question addresses the overall health status, based on the other six questions, scoring 0 to 10. The maximum score is 48 and represents the greatest symptom burden.[83]
- *Leiden Bother and Needs Questionnaire for patients with pituitary disease*: A self-rating questionnaire that compromises 26 items, scoring 0 to 4, and covering five domains (mood problems, negative illness perceptions, issues in sexual functioning, physical and cognitive complaints, and issues in social functioning).[84]

Domain-specific Patient-Reported Outcome Measures Relevant to Acromegaly

PROMs originally developed in other patient populations that measure specific dimensions are also relevant for patients with acromegaly, such as anxiety and depression symptoms (eg, HADS[85]), joint complaints (eg, Australian/Canadian Osteoarthritis Hand Index[86]), fatigue (eg, Multidimensional Fatigue Inventory-20[87]), cognitive functioning (eg, Cognitive Failure Questionnaire[88]), sleeping problems (eg, Epworth Sleepiness Scale[89]), sexual function (eg, Female Sexual Function Index[90]), or social situation (eg, Social Adjustment Scale[91,92]). These domain-specific PROMs assess domains at the level of symptom status and functional status as per the Wilson–Cleary model. One can also use domain-specific PROMs at the level of individual characteristics (eg, Beliefs about Medicine Questionnaire,[93] Brief Illness Perception Questionnaire,[94] or environmental characteristics [work role functioning questionnaire 2.0[95]]).

Generic Patient-Reported Outcome Measures

- *EuroQol 5 dimensions:* A self-rating questionnaire that compromises 6 items (5 multiple choice questions, scoring 1–3 and one visual analog scale, scoring 0–100) and covers five domains to assess the utility and health-related QoL.[96]
- *Short Form-36:* A non-disease-specific, self-rating questionnaire that compromises 36 items and covers eight domains (general health, vitality, physical functioning, bodily pain, physical role functioning, emotional role functioning, social role functioning, and mental health) which yield a physical component score and mental component score to assess health-related QoL. The ninth domain is the role–social component and is sometimes reported as well.[97]

Standardized Outcome Measures for Acromegaly

Scoring tools such as ACROmegaly Disease Activity Tool[98] and combining Signs and symptoms, Associated comorbidities, Growth hormone levels, IGF-1 levels, and Tumor profile[99] are useful instruments to assess overall disease activity. Both instruments combine clinician-observed outcomes (IGF-1 and GH levels, tumor status, associated comorbidities symptoms) with PROMs (patient-perceived health status). However, comprehensive PROMs are still lacking, especially to evaluate the efficacy of personalized medicine, which is receiving increasing attention in the treatment of acromegaly.[4,100] For example, the HADS, by paying attention to—and evaluating the treatment of psychopathological comorbidities (by either psychological or pharmaceutical approaches), may provide added value to the chronic care of patients with acromegaly with depressive symptoms or anxiety.

DETERMINANTS OF QUALITY OF LIFE

As previously described, determinants of general health perception and QoL can be categorized following the conceptual model of Wilson and Claery.[17] Based on the previous literature overview, we adapted this model for acromegaly with main causal relationships and mediating factors (**Fig. 1**). Factors contributing to impairments in QoL include higher GH and IGF-1 levels, GH deficiency after treatment, and having undergone conventional radiotherapy (biological and physiologic factors); pain (mainly arthropathy pain), anxiety, and depressive symptoms (symptom status); and impairments in cognitive functioning (functional status), and individual characteristics including older age at onset, female gender, and higher body mass index (BMI).[11–14,44,100,101]

The Contribution of Biochemical Outcome to Quality of Life

Following the Wilson and Cleary model, a cascade of improvement can be induced by the normalization of biological and physiologic variables.[17] In acromegaly, this could, for instance, be induced by controlling excess GH and/or IGF-1 levels. In a recent meta-analysis, including 53 intervention and cohort studies and 3667 acromegaly patients, it was reported that in most studies (n = 34, 64%), the improvement of PROMs was accompanied by a significant decrease in IGF-1 levels, both in the intervention

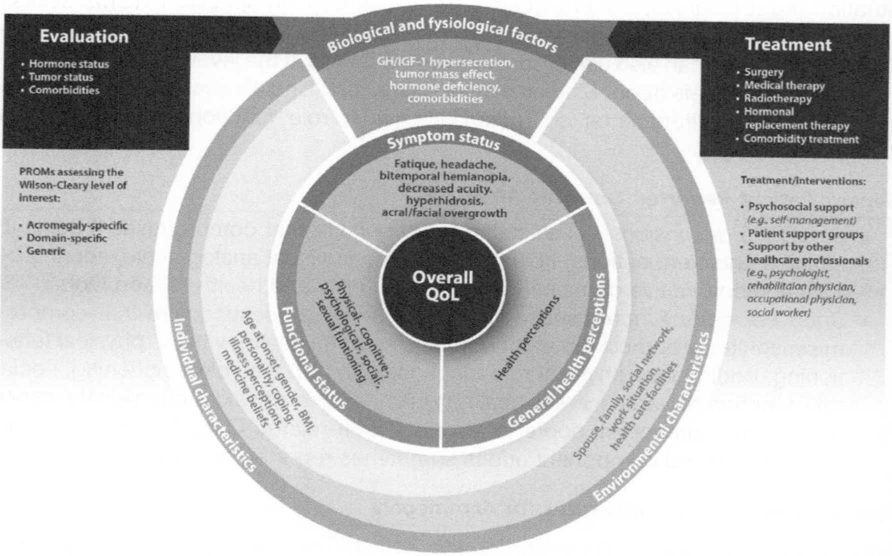

Fig. 1. A conceptual model for acromegaly including diagnostic and therapeutic interventions and the use of PROM based on the Wilson and Cleary model.[17]

(mean difference: −292 g/L, 95% CI -372 – −211) and cohort studies (mean difference: −326 g/L, 95% CI -496 – −157).[81] In 28 intervention studies, the improvement of PROMs was accompanied by a significant decrease in GH levels (mean difference: −10.7, 95% CI -13.2 – −8.3); however, this was not observed in cohort studies (mean difference: −1·6 g/L, 95% CI -4.7–1.5).[81]

Nevertheless, in the evaluation of the contribution of biochemical outcomes to QoL, one should take into account that the discrepancy between biochemical outcome and symptomatology in acromegaly is not straightforward, including the biopsychosocial factors mentioned above, and variable and tissue-specific GH and/or IGF-1 sensitivity.[100–109] In the same meta-analysis,[81] the authors also studied the differences between PROMs and conventional biochemical outcomes. In a third of the studies among patients with acromegaly (n = 18, 34%), discrepancies exist between PROMs and conventional biochemical outcomes (ie, both changed in opposite directions). The percentage of discrepant results was slightly higher among studies measuring QoL (38%) compared with studies measuring patients' symptoms (32%). In half of the studies with discrepant results ($n = 10$, 56%), biochemical outcomes overall improved with treatment, although QoL and patients' symptoms remained the same across most domains. No clear determinants of this dissociation were identified.

Next, the phenomenon called "extrahepatic acromegaly" may play a role in medically treated patients.[110] In addition to the suppression of GH secretion from the somatotroph tumor, somatostatin receptor ligands (SRLs) also suppress insulin secretion in the portal vein, which by itself downregulates hepatic IGF-1 production via GH receptors. Nevertheless, the GH action in the peripheral tissues (eg, white adipose tissue, bone, and kidney) remains unaltered and might still have acromegaly-inducing effects.[110] To put it another way, extrahepatic GH activity may remain elevated despite normal IGF-1 levels. If the addition of the GH-receptor antagonist pegvisomant could antagonize these extrahepatic GH actions in patients using first-generation or second-generation SRLs, one might observe an improvement of QoL in comparison with SRL monotherapy. Indeed, it has been shown previously that the addition of pegvisomant to the first-generation long-acting SRL therapy in acromegaly patients can improve GH-dependent parameters of QoL and patients' symptoms (eg, headache and soft-tissue swelling),[111] irrespective of the improved IGF-1 control. Data from intervention studies on other medical therapies were too limited to draw conclusions on the effects of these modalities on QoL.

RECOMMENDATIONS FOR THE MANAGEMENT OF ACROMEGALY

Optimal management of acromegaly by achieving biochemical control correlates with improvements in QoL, morbidity, functional outcome and health care-related costs, and reduced mortality risk, albeit not to the levels seen in the general population.[15] Although some comorbidities may be reversible after cure or disease control, many other complications could persist or even progress when the disease is controlled. In light of the incomplete reversibility of some comorbidities, optimal disease management seems to be crucial to prevent major side effects that may, in turn, lead to these premature comorbidities and impaired QoL. Therefore, in addition to normalizing GH and IGF-1 and achieving tumor volume control, if possible with preserving pituitary function, prompt diagnosis and treatment of acromegaly-associated comorbidities are critical to pursuing a good functional status, optimal QoL, and ensuring the best long-term outcome for this chronic illness.[4,80] There is a need to consider both IGF-1 and GH levels and PROMs to judge the status of control. Next, the model of Wilson and Cleary can be used to offer a holistic individualized approach and better understand variability in the outcome and other determinants of QoL.[17]

The patient perspective on their symptoms, functional status, and QoL is important to address during the care process and is ideally measured longitudinally and used for shared decision-making. Although the AcroQoL and the PASQ are acromegaly-specific and frequently used PROMs, the PASQ has not been validated (yet) in acromegaly or any other patient populations. Therefore, in accordance with the current consensus criteria, it is recommended to assess disease-specific QoL via the AcroQoL annually.[4] For clinical trials in patients with acromegaly, it is advised to use a disease-specific PROM (eg, AcroQoL or PASQ if validated for acromegaly), in combination with a generic QoL measure (eg, SF-36 if validated for acromegaly) and depending on the specific study aim, a domain-specific PROM.

A patient-centered approach, accounting for conventional biochemical outcomes, tumor control, comorbidities, treatment complications, and PROMs, should all be considered in treatment decisions.[9] PROMs have added value in guiding treatment decisions, in particular when patients are only partial responders to treatment. In patients with discrepant results between PROMs and conventional biochemical outcomes, PROMs have incremental value and should be incorporated in the evaluation of treatment efficacy.[112] Better markers of disease activity are still warranted to decrease this clinical burden. In general, it remains difficult to judge an effective treatment of acromegaly on biochemical outcome parameters alone, partly because every patient has an individual optimal hormonal setpoint[113] but also impairment in QoL may be caused by permanent damage, that is, unresponsive to treatment. In addition, extrahepatic GH activity[110] and hormonal oversubstitution or undersubstitution could be identified and corrected with PROMs. Therefore, both conventional biochemical outcomes and PROMs are pivotal to obtain a comprehensive view of disease activity.

Acromegaly is a rare condition with severe chronic multiorgan and multisystemic morbidities requiring life-long complex multidisciplinary treatment. The Pituitary Tumor Centers of Excellence[114] provides this multimodal management to achieve biochemical and tumor control as well as providing access for patients to a wide range of health care providers to diagnose, monitor, and treat acromegaly-associated comorbidities. A more integrated approach seems effective in treating comorbidities and improving patient-reported outcomes and is critical, as many patients do not achieve biochemical or tumor control and comorbidities, impairment in QoL may not remit even when full biochemical control is achieved.[114,115]

SUMMARY

Acromegaly has a substantial negative impact on QoL. A patient-centered approach should be considered in treatment decisions, integrating conventional biochemical outcomes, tumor control, comorbidities, treatment complications, and PROMs, including QoL measures.

CLINICS CARE POINTS

Recommendations for evaluating the effect of acromegaly on quality of life (QoL)

- A patient-centered approach, accounting for conventional biochemical outcomes, tumor control, comorbidities, treatment complications, and patient-reported outcome measures (PROMs), should all be considered in treatment decisions.

- The patient's perspective on their symptoms, functional status, and QoL is important to address during the care process and is ideally measured longitudinally and used for shared decision-making.
- In the light of the incomplete reversibility of some comorbidities, optimal disease management is crucial to prevent major side effects that may, in turn, lead to premature comorbidities and impaired QoL.

Areas where further research is needed

- Better markers of disease activity are still warranted to guide management decisions (eg, interventions and dose titration) to ultimately decrease the clinical burden in patients with acromegaly.
- Proper reporting of the use, analysis, and outcomes of validated and unvalidated generic and disease-specific PROMs in publications is needed to facilitate translation of the PROMs into clinical practice.
- Development of comprehensive PROMs in research, including a disease-specific PROM, in combination with a generic QoL measure, and depending on the specific study aim, a domain-specific PROM is needed. Likewise, further development of effective PROMs for use in clinical practice is needed.

DECLARATION OF INTEREST

The authors report no conflict of interest.

CONFLICT OF INTEREST

The authors declare that they have no conflict of interest.

FUNDING

This work did not receive any specific grant from any funding agency in the public, commercial, or non-profit sector.

REFERENCES

1. Sibeoni J, Manolios E, Verneuil L, et al. Patients' perspectives on acromegaly diagnostic delay: a qualitative study. Eur J Endocrinol 2019;180(6):339–52.
2. Colao A, Grasso LFS, Giustina A, et al. Acromegaly. Nat Rev Dis Primers 2019; 5(1):20.
3. Katznelson L, Laws ER Jr, Melmed S, et al. Acromegaly: an endocrine society clinical practice guideline. J Clin Endocrinol Metab 2014;99(11):3933–51.
4. Giustina A, Barkan A, Beckers A, et al. A Consensus on the Diagnosis and Treatment of Acromegaly Comorbidities: An Update. J Clin Endocrinol Metab 2020; 105(4):e937–46.
5. Sherlock M, Ayuk J, Tomlinson JW, et al. Mortality in patients with pituitary disease. Endocr Rev 2010;31(3):301–42.
6. Dekkers OM, Biermasz NR, Pereira AM, et al. Mortality in acromegaly: a meta-analysis. J Clin Endocrinol Metab 2008;93(1):61–7.
7. McCabe J, Ayuk J, Sherlock M. Treatment Factors That Influence Mortality in Acromegaly. Neuroendocrinology 2016;103(1):66–74.
8. Gadelha MR, Kasuki L, Lim DST, et al. Systemic Complications of Acromegaly and the Impact of the Current Treatment Landscape: An Update. Endocr Rev 2019;40(1):268–332.
9. Ben-Shlomo A, Sheppard MC, Stephens JM, et al. Clinical, quality of life, and economic value of acromegaly disease control. Pituitary 2011;14(3):284–94.

10. Christofides EA. Clinical importance of achieving biochemical control with medical therapy in adult patients with acromegaly. Patient Prefer Adherence 2016; 10:1217–25.
11. Andela CD, Scharloo M, Pereira AM, et al. Quality of life (QoL) impairments in patients with a pituitary adenoma: a systematic review of QoL studies. Pituitary 2015;18(5):752–76.
12. Tiemensma J, Kaptein AA, Pereira AM, et al. Affected illness perceptions and the association with impaired quality of life in patients with long-term remission of acromegaly. J Clin Endocrinol Metab 2011;96(11):3550–8.
13. Sievers C, Ising M, Pfister H, et al. Personality in patients with pituitary adenomas is characterized by increased anxiety-related traits: comparison of 70 acromegalic patients with patients with non-functioning pituitary adenomas and age- and gender-matched controls. Eur J Endocrinol 2009;160(3):367–73.
14. Webb SM, Badia X. Quality of Life in Acromegaly. Neuroendocrinology 2016; 103(1):106–11.
15. Whittington MD, Munoz KA, Whalen JD, et al. Economic and clinical burden of comorbidities among patients with acromegaly. Growth Horm IGF Res 2021;59: 101389.
16. U.S. Department of Health and Human Services FDA Center for Drug Evaluation and Research; U.S. Department of Health and Human Services FDA Center for Biologics Evaluation and Research; U.S. Department of Health and Human Services FDA Center for Devices and Radiological Health. Guidance for industry: patient-reported outcome measures: use in medical product development to support labeling claims: draft guidance. Health Qual LifeOutcomes 2006;4:79.
17. Wilson IB, Cleary PD. Linking clinical variables with health-related quality of life. A conceptual model of patient outcomes. JAMA 1995;273(1):59–65.
18. Carmichael JD, Broder MS, Cherepanov D, et al. The association between biochemical control and cardiovascular risk factors in acromegaly. BMC Endocr Disord 2017;17(1):15.
19. Fleseriu M, Barkan A, Del Pilar Schneider M, et al. Prevalence of comorbidities and concomitant medication use in acromegaly: analysis of real-world data from the United States. Pituitary 2022;25(2):296–307.
20. Maison P, Tropeano AI, Macquin-Mavier I, et al. Impact of somatostatin analogs on the heart in acromegaly: a metaanalysis. J Clin Endocrinol Metab 2007;92(5): 1743–7.
21. Pivonello R, Galderisi M, Auriemma RS, et al. Treatment with growth hormone receptor antagonist in acromegaly: effect on cardiac structure and performance. J Clin Endocrinol Metab 2007;92(2):476–82.
22. Claessen KM, Kroon HM, Pereira AM, et al. Progression of vertebral fractures despite long-term biochemical control of acromegaly: a prospective follow-up study. J Clin Endocrinol Metab 2013;98(12):4808–15.
23. Zhang Z, Li Q, He W, et al. The comprehensive impact on human body induced by resolution of growth hormone excess. Eur J Endocrinol 2018;178(4):365–75.
24. Chemla D, Attal P, Maione L, et al. Impact of successful treatment of acromegaly on overnight heart rate variability and sleep apnea. J Clin Endocrinol Metab 2014;99(8):2925–31.
25. Davi MV, Dalle Carbonare L, Giustina A, et al. Sleep apnoea syndrome is highly prevalent in acromegaly and only partially reversible after biochemical control of the disease. Eur J Endocrinol 2008;159(5):533–40.

26. Dal J, Leisner MZ, Hermansen K, et al. Cancer Incidence in Patients With Acromegaly: A Cohort Study and Meta-Analysis of the Literature. J Clin Endocrinol Metab 2018;103(6):2182–8.
27. Ritvonen E, Loyttyniemi E, Jaatinen P, et al. Mortality in acromegaly: a 20-year follow-up study. Endocr Relat Cancer 2016;23(6):469–80.
28. Maione L, Brue T, Beckers A, et al. Changes in the management and comorbidities of acromegaly over three decades: the French Acromegaly Registry. Eur J Endocrinol 2017;176(5):645–55.
29. Mercado M, Gonzalez B, Vargas G, et al. Successful mortality reduction and control of comorbidities in patients with acromegaly followed at a highly specialized multidisciplinary clinic. J Clin Endocrinol Metab 2014;99(12):4438–46.
30. Bolfi F, Neves AF, Boguszewski CL, et al. Mortality in acromegaly decreased in the last decade: a systematic review and meta-analysis. Eur J Endocrinol 2018; 179(1):59–71.
31. Brasso K, Ladelund S, Frederiksen BL, et al. Psychological distress following fecal occult blood test in colorectal cancer screening–a population-based study. Scand J Gastroenterol 2010;45(10):1211–6.
32. Miles A, Wardle J. Adverse psychological outcomes in colorectal cancer screening: does health anxiety play a role? Behav Res Ther 2006;44(8): 1117–27.
33. Bondanelli M, Ambrosio MR, degli Uberti EC. Pathogenesis and prevalence of hypertension in acromegaly. Pituitary 2001;4(4):239–49.
34. Alexopoulou O, Bex M, Kamenicky P, et al. Prevalence and risk factors of impaired glucose tolerance and diabetes mellitus at diagnosis of acromegaly: a study in 148 patients. Pituitary 2014;17(1):81–9.
35. Petrossians P, Daly AF, Natchev E, et al. Acromegaly at diagnosis in 3173 patients from the Liege Acromegaly Survey (LAS) Database. Endocr Relat Cancer 2017;24(10):505–18.
36. Hannon AM, Thompson CJ, Sherlock M. Diabetes in Patients With Acromegaly. Curr Diab Rep 2017;17(2):8.
37. Colao A, Baldelli R, Marzullo P, et al. Systemic hypertension and impaired glucose tolerance are independently correlated to the severity of the acromegalic cardiomyopathy. J Clin Endocrinol Metab 2000;85(1):193–9.
38. Holdaway IM, Rajasoorya RC, Gamble GD. Factors influencing mortality in acromegaly. J Clin Endocrinol Metab 2004;89(2):667–74.
39. Kauppinen-Makelin R, Sane T, Sintonen H, et al. Quality of life in treated patients with acromegaly. J Clin Endocrinol Metab 2006;91(10):3891–6.
40. Tseng FY, Huang TS, Lin JD, et al. A registry of acromegaly patients and one year following up in Taiwan. J Formos Med Assoc 2019;118(10):1430–7.
41. Romijn JA, Smit JW, Lamberts SW. Intrinsic imperfections of endocrine replacement therapy. Eur J Endocrinol 2003;149(2):91–7.
42. Mazziotti G, Formenti AM, Frara S, et al. MANAGEMENT OF ENDOCRINE DISEASE: Risk of overtreatment in patients with adrenal insufficiency: current and emerging aspects. Eur J Endocrinol 2017;177(5):R231–48.
43. Claessen K, Andela CD, Biermasz NR, et al. Clinical Unmet Needs in the Treatment of Adrenal Crisis: Importance of the Patient's Perspective. Front Endocrinol (Lausanne) 2021;12:701365.
44. Wexler T, Gunnell L, Omer Z, et al. Growth hormone deficiency is associated with decreased quality of life in patients with prior acromegaly. J Clin Endocrinol Metab 2009;94(7):2471–7.

45. Katznelson L, Kleinberg D, Vance ML, et al. Hypogonadism in patients with acromegaly: data from the multi-centre acromegaly registry pilot study. Clin Endocrinol (Oxf) 2001;54(2):183–8.
46. Annamalai AK, Webb A, Kandasamy N, et al. A comprehensive study of clinical, biochemical, radiological, vascular, cardiac, and sleep parameters in an unselected cohort of patients with acromegaly undergoing presurgical somatostatin receptor ligand therapy. J Clin Endocrinol Metab 2013;98(3):1040–50.
47. Kuhn E, Maione L, Bouchachi A, et al. Long-term effects of pegvisomant on comorbidities in patients with acromegaly: a retrospective single-center study. Eur J Endocrinol 2015;173(5):693–702.
48. Guo X, Gao L, Zhao Y, et al. Characteristics of the upper respiratory tract in patients with acromegaly and correlations with obstructive sleep apnoea/hypopnea syndrome. Sleep Med 2018;48:27–34.
49. Dostalova S, Sonka K, Smahel Z, et al. Craniofacial abnormalities and their relevance for sleep apnoea syndrome aetiopathogenesis in acromegaly. Eur J Endocrinol 2001;144(5):491–7.
50. Bradley TD, Floras JS. Obstructive sleep apnoea and its cardiovascular consequences. Lancet 2009;373(9657):82–93.
51. Wennberg A, Lorusso R, Dassie F, et al. Sleep disorders and cognitive dysfunction in acromegaly. Endocrine 2019;66(3):634–41.
52. Celik O, Kadioglu P. Quality of life in female patients with acromegaly. J Endocrinol Invest 2013;36(6):412–6.
53. Romijn JA. Pituitary diseases and sleep disorders. Curr Opin Endocrinol Diabetes Obes 2016;23(4):345–51.
54. Attal P, Chanson P. Endocrine aspects of obstructive sleep apnea. J Clin Endocrinol Metab 2010;95(2):483–95.
55. Mazziotti G, Maffezzoni F, Frara S, et al. Acromegalic osteopathy. Pituitary 2017;20(1):63–9.
56. Claessen KM, Ramautar SR, Pereira AM, et al. Progression of acromegalic arthropathy despite long-term biochemical control: a prospective, radiological study. Eur J Endocrinol 2012;167(2):235–44.
57. Pelsma ICM, Biermasz NR, van Furth WR, et al. Progression of acromegalic arthropathy in long-term controlled acromegaly patients: 9 years of longitudinal follow-up. J Clin Endocrinol Metab 2021;106(1):188–200.
58. Mazziotti G, Lania AGA, Canalis E. MANAGEMENT OF ENDOCRINE DISEASE: Bone disorders associated with acromegaly: mechanisms and treatment. Eur J Endocrinol 2019;181(2):R45–56.
59. Claessen KM, Mazziotti G, Biermasz NR, et al. Bone and Joint Disorders in Acromegaly. Neuroendocrinology 2016;103(1):86–95.
60. Cellini M, Biamonte E, Mazza M, et al. Vertebral Fractures Associated with Spinal Sagittal Imbalance and Quality of Life in Acromegaly: A Radiographic Study with EOS 2D/3D Technology. Neuroendocrinology 2021;111(8):775–85.
61. Wassenaar MJ, Biermasz NR, van Duinen N, et al. High prevalence of arthropathy, according to the definitions of radiological and clinical osteoarthritis, in patients with long-term cure of acromegaly: a case-control study. Eur J Endocrinol 2009;160(3):357–65.
62. Mazziotti G, Battista C, Maffezzoni F, et al. Treatment of Acromegalic Osteopathy in Real-life Clinical Practice: The BAAC (Bone Active Drugs in Acromegaly) Study. J Clin Endocrinol Metab 2020;105(9):e3285–92.
63. Claessen KMJA, Appelman-Dijkstra NM, Biermasz NR. Osteoporosis and arthropathy in functioning pituitary tumors. In: Honegger J, Reincke M,

Petersenn S, editors. Pituitary Tumors. A Comprehensive and Interdisciplinary Approach. Academic Press; 2021. p. 617–37.
64. Du F, Chen Q, Wang X, et al. Long-term facial changes and clinical correlations in patients with treated acromegaly: a cohort study. Eur J Endocrinol 2021; 184(2):231–41.
65. Wagenmakers MA, Roerink SH, Maal TJ, et al. Three-dimensional facial analysis in acromegaly: a novel tool to quantify craniofacial characteristics after long-term remission. Pituitary 2015;18(1):126–34.
66. Hoevenaren IA, Wagenmakers MA, Roerink SH, et al. Three-dimensional soft tissue analysis of the hand: a novel method to investigate effects of acromegaly. Eur J Plast Surg 2016;39(6):429–34.
67. Imran SA, Tiemensma J, Kaiser SM, et al. Morphometric changes correlate with poor psychological outcomes in patients with acromegaly. Eur J Endocrinol 2016;174(1):41–50.
68. Wolters TLC, Roerink S, Drenthen LCA, et al. Voice Characteristics in Patients with Acromegaly during Treatment. J Voice 2021;35(6):932 e13–e27.
69. Tiemensma J, Biermasz NR, van der Mast RC, et al. Increased psychopathology and maladaptive personality traits, but normal cognitive functioning, in patients after long-term cure of acromegaly. J Clin Endocrinol Metab 2010;95(12): E392–402.
70. Pertichetti M, Serioli S, Belotti F, et al. Pituitary adenomas and neuropsychological status: a systematic literature review. Neurosurg Rev 2020;43(4):1065–78.
71. Sievers C, Samann PG, Pfister H, et al. Cognitive function in acromegaly: description and brain volumetric correlates. Pituitary 2012;15(3):350–7.
72. Yedinak CG, Fleseriu M. Self-perception of cognitive function among patients with active acromegaly, controlled acromegaly, and non-functional pituitary adenoma: a pilot study. Endocrine 2014;46(3):585–93.
73. Pereira AM, Tiemensma J, Romijn JA, et al. Cognitive impairment and psychopathology in patients with pituitary diseases. Neth J Med 2012;70(6):255–60.
74. Lobatto DJ, Steffens ANV, Zamanipoor Najafabadi AH, et al. Work disability and its determinants in patients with pituitary tumor-related disease. Pituitary 2018; 21(6):593–604.
75. Andela CD, Niemeijer ND, Scharloo M, et al. Towards a better quality of life (QoL) for patients with pituitary diseases: results from a focus group study exploring QoL. Pituitary 2015;18(1):86–100.
76. Andela CD, Tiemensma J, Kaptein AA, et al. The partner's perspective of the impact of pituitary disease: Looking beyond the patient. J Health Psychol 2019;24(12):1687–97.
77. Celik O, Hatipoglu E, Akhan SE, et al. Acromegaly is associated with higher frequency of female sexual dysfunction: experience of a single center. Endocr J 2013;60(6):753–61.
78. Andela CD, Biermasz NR, Kaptein AA, et al. More concerns and stronger beliefs about the necessity of medication in patients with acromegaly are associated with negative illness perceptions and impairment in quality of life. Growth Horm IGF Res 2015;25(5):219–26.
79. Tiemensma J, Kaptein AA, Pereira AM, et al. Coping strategies in patients after treatment for functioning or nonfunctioning pituitary adenomas. J Clin Endocrinol Metab 2011;96(4):964–71.
80. Melmed S, Bronstein MD, Chanson P, et al. A Consensus Statement on acromegaly therapeutic outcomes. Nat Rev Endocrinol 2018;14(9):552–61.

81. van der Meulen M, Zamanipoor Najafabadi AH, Broersen LHA, et al. State of the art of patient-reported outcomes in acromegaly or GH deficiency: a systematic review and meta-analysis. J Clin Endocrinol Metab 2021;107(5):1225–38.
82. Webb SM, Prieto L, Badia X, et al. Acromegaly Quality of Life Questionnaire (ACROQOL) a new health-related quality of life questionnaire for patients with acromegaly: development and psychometric properties. Clin Endocrinol (Oxf) 2002;57(2):251–8.
83. Trainer PJ, Drake WM, Katznelson L, et al. Treatment of acromegaly with the growth hormone-receptor antagonist pegvisomant. N Engl J Med 2000; 342(16):1171–7.
84. Andela CD, Scharloo M, Ramondt S, et al. The development and validation of the Leiden Bother and Needs Questionnaire for patients with pituitary disease: the LBNQ-Pituitary. Pituitary 2016;19(3):293–302.
85. Zigmond AS, Snaith RP. The hospital anxiety and depression scale. Acta Psychiatr Scand 1983;67(6):361–70.
86. Bellamy N, Campbell J, Haraoui B, et al. Dimensionality and clinical importance of pain and disability in hand osteoarthritis: Development of the Australian/Canadian (AUSCAN) Osteoarthritis Hand Index. Osteoarthritis Cartilage 2002; 10(11):855–62.
87. Smets EM, Garssen B, Bonke B, et al. The Multidimensional Fatigue Inventory (MFI) psychometric qualities of an instrument to assess fatigue. J Psychosom Res 1995;39(3):315–25.
88. Broadbent DE, Cooper PF, FitzGerald P, et al. The Cognitive Failures Questionnaire (CFQ) and its correlates. Br J Clin Psychol 1982;21(1):1–16.
89. Johns MW. A new method for measuring daytime sleepiness: the Epworth sleepiness scale. Sleep 1991;14(6):540–5.
90. Rosen R, Brown C, Heiman J, et al. The Female Sexual Function Index (FSFI): a multidimensional self-report instrument for the assessment of female sexual function. J Sex Marital Ther 2000;26(2):191–208.
91. Weissman MM, Bothwell S. Assessment of social adjustment by patient self-report. Arch Gen Psychiatry 1976;33(9):1111–5.
92. Cooper P, Osborn M, Gath D, et al. Evaluation of a modified self-report measure of social adjustment. Br J Psychiatry 1982;141:68–75.
93. Horne R, Weinman J, Hankins M. The beliefs about medicines questionnaire: The development and evaluation of a new method for assessing the cognitive representation of medication. Psychol Health 1999;14(1):1–24.
94. Broadbent E, Petrie KJ, Main J, et al. The brief illness perception questionnaire. J Psychosom Res 2006;60(6):631–7.
95. Abma FI, van der Klink JJ, Bultmann U. The work role functioning questionnaire 2.0 (Dutch version): examination of its reliability, validity and responsiveness in the general working population. J Occup Rehabil 2013;23(1):135–47.
96. EuroQol G. EuroQol–a new facility for the measurement of health-related quality of life. Health Policy 1990;16(3):199–208.
97. Ware JE Jr, Sherbourne CD. The MOS 36-item short-form health survey (SF-36). I. Conceptual framework and item selection. Med Care 1992;30(6):473–83.
98. van der Lely AJ, Gomez R, Pleil A, et al. Development of ACRODAT((R)), a new software medical device to assess disease activity in patients with acromegaly. Pituitary 2017;20(6):692–701.
99. Giustina A, Bevan JS, Bronstein MD, et al. SAGIT(R): clinician-reported outcome instrument for managing acromegaly in clinical practice–development and results from a pilot study. Pituitary 2016;19(1):39–49.

100. Geraedts VJ, Andela CD, Stalla GK, et al. Predictors of Quality of Life in Acromegaly: No Consensus on Biochemical Parameters. Front Endocrinol (Lausanne) 2017;8:40.
101. Biermasz NR, van Thiel SW, Pereira AM, et al. Decreased quality of life in patients with acromegaly despite long-term cure of growth hormone excess. J Clin Endocrinol Metab 2004;89(11):5369–76.
102. Kyriakakis N, Lynch J, Gilbey SG, et al. Impaired quality of life in patients with treated acromegaly despite long-term biochemically stable disease: Results from a 5-years prospective study. Clin Endocrinol (Oxf) 2017;86(6):806–15.
103. Baum HB, Katznelson L, Sherman JC, et al. Effects of physiological growth hormone (GH) therapy on cognition and quality of life in patients with adult-onset GH deficiency. J Clin Endocrinol Metab 1998;83(9):3184–9.
104. Hua SC, Yan YH, Chang TC. Associations of remission status and lanreotide treatment with quality of life in patients with treated acromegaly. Eur J Endocrinol 2006;155(6):831–7.
105. Biermasz NR, Pereira AM, Smit JW, et al. Morbidity after long-term remission for acromegaly: persisting joint-related complaints cause reduced quality of life. J Clin Endocrinol Metab 2005;90(5):2731–9.
106. Bonapart IE, van Domburg R, ten Have SMTH, et al. The 'bio-assay'quality of life might be a better marker of disease activity in acromegalic patients than serum total IGF-I concentrations. Eur J Endocrinol 2005;152(2):217–24.
107. Rowles SV, Prieto L, Badia X, et al. Quality of life (QOL) in patients with acromegaly is severely impaired: use of a novel measure of QOL: acromegaly quality of life questionnaire. J Clin Endocrinol Metab 2005;90(6):3337–41.
108. Coopmans EC, El-Sayed N, Frystyk J, et al. Soluble Klotho: a possible predictor of quality of life in acromegaly patients. Endocrine 2020;69(1):165–74.
109. Broersen LHA, Zamanipoor Najafabadi AH, Pereira AM, et al. Improvement in Symptoms and Health-Related Quality of Life in Acromegaly Patients: A Systematic Review and Meta-Analysis. J Clin Endocrinol Metab 2021;106(2):577–87.
110. Neggers SJ, Kopchick JJ, Jorgensen JO, et al. Hypothesis: Extra-hepatic acromegaly: a new paradigm? Eur J Endocrinol 2011;164(1):11–6.
111. Neggers SJCMM, van Aken MO, de Herder WW, et al. Quality of Life in Acromegalic Patients during Long-Term Somatostatin Analog Treatment with and without Pegvisomant. J Clin Endocrinol Metab 2008;93(10):3853–9.
112. Zeinalizadeh M, Habibi Z, Fernandez-Miranda JC, et al. Discordance between growth hormone and insulin-like growth factor-1 after pituitary surgery forA acromegaly: a stepwise approach and management. Pituitary 2015;18(1):48–59.
113. Biermasz NR, Pereira AM, Frolich M, et al. Octreotide represses secretory-burst mass and nonpulsatile secretion but does not restore event frequency or orderly GH secretion in acromegaly. Am J Physiol Endocrinol Metab 2004;286(1): E25–30.
114. Casanueva FF, Barkan AL, Buchfelder M, et al. Criteria for the definition of Pituitary Tumor Centers of Excellence (PTCOE): A Pituitary Society Statement. Pituitary 2017;20(5):489–98.
115. Melmed S. Pituitary Medicine From Discovery to Patient-Focused Outcomes. J Clin Endocrinol Metab 2016;101(3):769–77.

Patient-Reported Outcomes in Endoscopic Endonasal Skull Base Surgery

Rabih Bou-Nassif, MD[a,b], Zaki Abou-Mrad, MD[a,b], Tarek Y. El Ahmadieh, MD[a,b], Viviane Tabar, MD[a,b], Marc A. Cohen, MD[b,c,*]

KEYWORDS

- Patient-reported outcomes (PROs) • Pituitary surgery
- Endoscopic endonasal skull base surgery (EESBS)
- Patient-reported outcome measures (PROMs)

KEY POINTS

- Patient-reported outcomes (PROs) provide valuable data in assessing endoscopic skull base surgery outcomes.
- PROs in skull base surgery have evolved from those evaluating objective and subjective smell dysfunction to more complex assessments of multiple areas of concern to the patient.
- There is now a variety of tools used to capture skull base surgery PROs.
- PROs facilitate and standardize the communication between the patient and treating physicians and may lead to more personalized approaches.
- Because this field is still in its infancy, extensive research is needed to capture the influence of surgical nuances on patients due to the heterogeneity of these tumors.

INTRODUCTION

During the past several decades, transsphenoidal surgery has been increasingly used to gain access to various skull base lesions, including sellar and suprasellar tumors, achieving good clinical and oncologic outcomes. Little attention has traditionally been given to the functional outcome, quality of life (QoL), and patient feedback related to a chosen treatment approach. With the current advances in endoscopic optical imaging technology and surgical precision, which have radically lowered the

[a] Department of Neurosurgery, Memorial Sloan Kettering Cancer Center, 1275 York Avenue, New York, NY 10065, USA; [b] Pituitary and Skull Base Tumor Program, Memorial Sloan Kettering Cancer Center, 1275 York Avenue, New York, NY 10065, USA; [c] Department of Surgery, Head and Neck Service, Memorial Sloan Kettering Cancer Center, 1275 York Avenue, New York, NY 10065, USA
* Corresponding author. Pituitary and Skull Base Tumor Program, Memorial Sloan Kettering Cancer Center, 1275 York Avenue, New York, NY 10065.
E-mail address: cohenm2@mskcc.org

Endocrinol Metab Clin N Am 51 (2022) 727–739
https://doi.org/10.1016/j.ecl.2022.04.005

perioperative morbidity associated with skull base surgery,[1–3] a shift toward a higher focus on patient-reported outcomes (PROs) has been recently observed. This shift has become imperative in an era of growing patient-centric approach to medical and surgical conditions. It is now critical to ensure that the offered treatment plan and approach align with the patient's preferences and expectations, in addition to the surgeon's best clinical judgment and experience.

PROs represent a view that reflects the patient's own thoughts and perspective on their condition and the management options, without input or interpretations from the surgeon. The patient's viewpoint is particularly important when distinguishing between 2 or more medically or surgically equivalent treatment strategies or procedures. One management plan might be preferred over the other based on their personal beliefs, their occupation, their short-term and long-term wants and needs, their expectations of the procedure, and their perception and tolerance of pain. Therefore, having PRO data enables patients the opportunity to learn from the experiences and perspectives of other patients who have been through a similar condition and/or a treatment approach, and allows patients to predict and evaluate the evolution of their own outcomes through different treatment phases. This input empowers patients to become active participants in the decision-making process at different stages of their care.

Understanding the advantages and disadvantages of skull base surgery from a patient's perspective is extremely valuable and requires an assessment of relevant PROs. An in-depth PRO evaluation requires specific validated tools and scoring systems, namely the patient-reported outcome measurement (PROM) tools. In this review, we discuss the currently available skull-base-related PROs, the assessment tools used to capture them, and the future trends of this important topic that is in its infancy.

REVIEW OF THE LITERATURE

PubMed, Scopus, Web-of-Science, and Cochrane were searched from database inception to January 22, 2022 using the following Medical Subject Headings (MeSH) terms: PROs, skull base surgery, endoscopy, and pituitary. Studies were included if they investigated PROs using PROM tools in patients who underwent skull base surgery. Two authors independently screened the titles and abstracts of all articles, and then assessed full texts of studies meeting the inclusion criteria. Disagreements were solved by a third author. The references of each article were searched to retrieve additional relevant studies.

PATIENT-REPORTED OUTCOMES AND PATIENT-REPORTED OUTCOME MEASUREMENTS

PROs constitute the data that is directly reported by the patient, without any interpretation, influence, or modification by a clinician. The PROMs are the questionnaires and objective scores used to collect the PROs. These questionnaires are directed at the patients themselves using understandable language to assess the way patients perceive their illness, the performed treatment, and specific situations encountered along the clinical course. Therefore, PROs are most informative when captured at different stages of the disease and the treatment. The implementation of PROs and PROMs in endoscopic skull base surgery remains in its infancy and, for the most part, borrows tools validated in sinonasal surgery because of the anatomic relation and technical similarities between the 2 disciplines. More recently, this effort has gained momentum because of the digital transformation in medicine, which has become more pronounced following the COVID pandemic.[4] The patient's participation has become easier and more efficient because completing a questionnaire at one's own comfort and timing makes it less of a burden. Each test has a particular domain of interest that will be discussed in detail in each section.

The Minimal Clinically Important Difference

Every tool used in the evaluation of clinical scenarios requires a clear assessment. The tools used in PROs to measure physiologic variables are evaluated by 2 essential criteria. The first is the reliability of the instrument, that is, whether it yields the same results when repeated in a stable environment. The second is the validity of the test, that is, whether it measures what it is claimed to measure. In addition to these 2 criteria, an important variable is the responsiveness of a test. Tools can be highly reliable yet minimally responsive to change, and vice versa. When using QoL measurement tools, responsiveness to change is of high importance, especially because change can be clinically relevant over time. Guyatt and colleagues[5] established the minimal clinically important difference (MCID) to evaluate instruments designed to measure change over time. The MCID was established as an effective index to evaluate the clinical meaningfulness of QoL score change.[6] It is directly related to sample size and therefore can be used to predetermine the necessary size of a clinical trial sample. MCID can be calculated by finding the smallest change in score that would be reported as a noticeable difference by the patient.[7,8]

Specific Tools

There has been an evolution in metrics that have been used to assess PROs in patients undergoing open and endoscopic skull base surgery. The current tools may be thought of as deriving from the initial assessment of objective and subjective olfactory dysfunction with progression to PROs in chronic sinusitis and finally the integration of these metrics for those undergoing skull base surgery for malignancy and benign conditions, including pituitary surgery.

Olfaction and Endoscopic Endonasal Skull Base Surgery

Olfaction is of high importance in the patient's daily life and can influence QoL. A decreased sense of smell can influence the patients' ability to enjoy food and beverages and their ability to detect dangerous smells such as smoke or gas leaks. It is also extremely important and required for some patient occupations for example, cooks. Further, olfaction impairment has been associated with an increased risk of depression. This can be directly related either to a decrease in the patients' QoL from the inability to enjoy food and participate in social events or to an imbalanced emotional control secondary to a reduced olfactory bulb input via the amygdala into the limbic circuit.[9]

Olfactory dysfunction after endoscopic endonasal skull base surgery may occur due to direct damage to the posterior septal olfactory mucosa or due to airflow modification around the olfactory mucosa caused by an anatomic modification after surgery.[10] Patient self-assessment of olfactory dysfunction was shown to lack reliability.[11] To that effect, several tests have been described for quantification and evaluation of the olfactory dysfunction. Comparison between endoscopic and microscopic transsphenoidal approaches was made possible, with a slightly better, although statistically insignificant improvement in olfactory outcomes in the endoscopic approach. This was justified by Kahilogullari and colleagues[12] to be caused by an unbalanced force applied during microscopic surgery on the posterior olfactory groove and displacement of the bony septum laterally, resulting in a laceration of the submucosal layers and synechia formation, which may cause anosmia.

To prevent cerebrospinal fluid leaks, a nasoseptal flap can be harvested and used to cover defects in the skull base. When referring to the nasoseptal flap, this is the Hadad-Bassagasteguy (HB) flap, which is a vascularized mucoperichondrial and mucoperiosteal axial pattern flap based on the posterior branch of the sphenopalatine artery.[13] The rescue flap is a modification of the standard approach, which involves a posterior superior septectomy with preservation of the nasoseptal flap pedicle for use if needed after the procedure is complete or in a separate intervention.[14] The rescue flap was reported to cause less olfactory dysfunction than the HB flap but more than when no flap was performed (14.4% vs 3%).[15]

Specific Olfactory Measures

The University of Pennsylvania Smell Identification Test (UPSIT) was developed by Doty and colleagues[16] in 1984 to accurately evaluate and diagnose olfactory dysfunction complaints. The test can be self-administered and uses a booklet with odor-releasing scratching areas. The authors stated that the test reliably detects sensitive aspects of olfaction impairment as well as parosmias. The UPSIT was used by Pucinelli and colleagues[17] to prove that olfactory perception at 1-year follow-up after an endonasal approach for skull base surgery was comparable between cold knife and cautery upper septal limb incisions. Different timepoints have also shown comparable outcomes. Tam and colleagues[15] showed deteriorated UPSIT scores 6 months after endonasal endoscopic skull base surgery. Doty and colleagues[18] described the 12-item Cross-Cultural Smell Identification Test (CC-SIT), which was based on items from the UPSIT. They removed the odors that were considered less familiar to patients from North American, European, South American, and Asian cultures. The CC-SIT was then tested and found comparable to the UPSIT. The authors concluded that the test was a reliable tool for a quick self-assessment of olfactory function.

Developed by Kobal and colleagues,[19] the Sniffin' Sticks test is widely used for screening olfactory dysfunction using 7 different odors with 4 multiple-choice answers. Its reliability and ease of application has made this test one of the top tests used for screening of olfaction. It is often used for validation of newer tests.[20] The butanol threshold test (BTT) uses n-butyl alcohol (1-butanol), which is an odorant widely used mainly because of its low toxicity, water solubility, and neutral odor quality. The BTT is also used as a component of the Connecticut Chemosensory Clinical Research Center test.[21]

Olfactory Only Patient-Reported Outcomes

Assessment of self-reported olfactory functioning and olfaction related quality of life

The assessment of self-reported olfactory functioning and olfaction-related QoL (ASOF) test is a 12-item questionnaire developed by Pusswald and colleagues[20] in 2012. It assesses 3 domains: the 1-item subjective olfactory capability scale, the 5-item self-reported capability of perceiving specific odors scale, and the 6-item olfactory-related quality of life scale. Validation of the test was performed by comparing healthy, olfactory-intact individuals with olfaction-impaired individuals, after confirmation by the Sniffin' Sticks test.

Raikundalia and colleagues used the ASOF as a first olfactory-specific QoL questionnaire in endoscopic endonasal skull base surgery.[22] They concluded that the ASOF would serve as a useful complementary tool in assessing olfaction after endoscopic endonasal skull base surgery but noted a discordance between the ASOF and the UPSIT. Although the UPSIT was more sensitive to age (older age was associated with poorer scores after surgery), the ASOF demonstrated poorer scores after bigger tumoral size surgery. This suggests that more focus should be invested in research in subjective olfactory-related QoL to better assess olfactory dysfunction and its influence on QoL after endoscopic skull base surgery.

Patient-Reported Outcome Measures Including More Than Olfaction

The 22-item sino-nasal outcome test

The 22-item sino-nasal outcome test (SNOT-22) consists of 22 questions on a Likert scale, each ranging from 0 to 5, with a maximal total score of 110. A higher score indicates more severe impairment of sinonasal QoL.[23] A patient with a score lower than 20 is considered asymptomatic.[24] The SNOT-22 was developed as a modification of the preexisting SNOT-20, which was derived from the Rhino-Sinusitis Outcome Measure-31, by adding 2 measurements pertaining to nasal blockage and the loss of taste and smell. The SNOT-22 has been validated in the evaluation of the patient QoL in chronic sinusitis. This has led to its utilization in several studies that evaluated patient QoL after endoscopic skull base surgery,[25–28] despite the existence of skull base-specific metrics in other assessment tools.[29,30]

A multicenter prospective trial assessed the validity of SNOT-22 in pituitary surgery in 2021.[31] QoL was evaluated using both SNOT-22 and the Anterior Skull Base Nasal Inventory-12 (ASK Nasal-12; a validated score in endonasal skull base surgery that will be discussed in the subheading "The Anterior Skull Base Nasal Inventory-12") in 113 patients with pituitary tumors treated endoscopically. This study showed concurrent validity between the 2 tests, which led the authors to conclude that the SNOT-22 is valid for assessing endoscopic pituitary surgery patients. However, only 11 out of the 22 items in the SNOT-22 changed 2 weeks after surgery, suggesting that the SNOT-22 may not be highly sensitive to PRO changes after endoscopic pituitary surgery, and thus not ideal for this patient population.

It is important to note that in contrast to patients undergoing intervention for sinusitis, endoscopic skull base surgery patients typically have fewer or no sinonasal complaints preoperatively but usually do experience discomfort in the immediate postoperative period. These symptoms, mainly nasal crusting and impaired olfaction, in some cases can take months to regress.[32] The use of a vascularized nasoseptal flap has also been linked to some adverse olfactory outcomes[17] in addition to other side effects and complications, notably septal cartilage necrosis, soft tissue damage, and in some cases flap necrosis.[33,34] Overall, the SNOT-22 can reliably assess sinonasal symptoms. It evaluates olfactory and neurocognitive outcomes after surgery. When used for assessing QoL outcomes of endoscopic endonasal skull base surgery, the SNOT-22 showed that patients usually regain their baseline scores 3 months after surgery. After that point, some patients show improvements beyond their baseline, reaching their peak level of improvement 1 year postoperatively.[35]

The Sino-Nasal Outcome Test for Neurosurgery

The Sino-Nasal Outcome Test for Neurosurgery (SNOT-NC) was derived from the SNOT-22 by Ahmadipour and colleagues[36] as a more neurosurgically oriented test capable of capturing the nasal discomfort outcome in patients who underwent endonasal transsphenoidal surgery for skull base lesions. The SNOT-NC is a 23-item score covering the domains of nasal discomfort, sleep and productivity issues, ear or head discomfort, and visual and olfactory impairment. The authors of this PROM used the Short Form-36 life quality questionnaire (a general health-related QoL assessment tool) and the Sniffin' Sticks test to evaluate its convergent and divergent validity. The study included 102 consecutive patients with sellar lesions who were treated through an endoscopic transsphenoidal approach. The authors found significant association between the SNOT-NC and a wide array of nasal symptoms by examining convergent and divergent validity.

They concluded that this test is a valid, reliable, and sensitive measure to assess the patient's nasal discomfort after endoscopic skull base surgery. Although there is a lot of promise with this measure, the test–retest reliability of this tool is yet to be established. In addition, this tool is currently only available in the German language.

The anterior skull base questionnaire

The anterior skull base questionnaire (ASBQ) was developed by Gil and colleagues[30] in 2004 to evaluate patient QoL after resection of anterior skull base tumors. Their initial series included 35 patients who were treated using the subcranial approach to the anterior skull base at least 3 months before the initiation of the study. The time between the surgery and the questionnaire completion ranged from 4 to 72 months. Their final questionnaire was reduced to 35 items from an initial 80-item list, following 2 testing phases and factor analyses with varimax rotation. The 6 domains evaluated by the ASBQ are performance, physical function, energy and vitality, pain, specific symptoms (such as smell, taste, appearance, epiphora, nasal secretions, and visual disturbances), and influence on emotions. Patients aged older than 60 years had poorer scores in the performance and physical function domains when compared with younger patients. Patients with malignant neoplasms had lower scores in the specific symptoms, influence on emotions, physical function, and performance domains in comparison with patients who had a benign tumor. Radiotherapy was associated with poorer outcomes in the specific symptoms and influence on emotions domains. Patients with comorbidities defined by the Charlson Comorbidity Index had poorer physical function outcomes. After finalizing their questionnaire, the authors evaluated it in 12 additional prospective patients, immediately before surgery, and again 5 to 6 months after surgery. The authors confirmed poorer reported outcomes in patients with malignancy compared with patients with a benign tumor. They concluded that the questionnaire was sufficiently reliable in evaluating QoL after skull base tumor resection. Caution should be used the generalizability of these early findings as these findings were seen in patients with sinonasal malignancies.

The MCID of the ASBQ was later reported to range between 8% and 12% reduction in QoL score.[8] Low QoL scores were associated with malignancy and the early postoperative period (<6 months). In addition, the type of surgical approach also showed clinically significant differences with endoscopic endonasal skull base surgery being associated with higher QoL scores compared with the subcranial approach, especially in the physical function and influence on emotions domains.

The Skull Base Inventory

The skull base inventory (SBI) was developed by de Almeida and colleagues[37] as a disease-specific QoL instrument, aimed for patients with anterior and central skull base pathologic condition. A chart review of 138 patients who underwent skull base surgery was performed, for which 5 experts rated physical items and domains. A systematic review of the literature was then performed, and 34 patients were recruited into 8 focus groups. This initial item screening yielded 77 items. Each of the elements was rated and items were reduced to a final list of 41 items covering cognitive, endocrine, nasal, neurologic, and visual domains. A preliminary cross-sectional reliability and validity of this instrument was established in a later study.[38]

A multicentric study was published in 2020 that aimed to prospectively assess the psychometric properties of the SBI.[39] Five centers participated in this study, with a total of 187 patients undergoing surgery for an anterior or central skull base lesion, including 121 patients by an endoscopic approach. A strong correlation between SBI and ASBQ scores ($r = 0.810–0.869$, $P < .001$) helped prove concurrent validity.

The MCID of the SBI was found to be 6.0. The internal consistency and test–retest at 12 months and 12 months plus 2 weeks were excellent (Cronbach's alpha = 0.95 and intraclass correlation > 0.90, respectively). The authors concluded that the SBI questionnaire is a reliable and valid tool for QoL assessment in patients undergoing open and endoscopic anterior and central skull base surgery. This validated tool is frequently used for patients undergoing transsphenoidal surgery.

The Anterior Skull Base Nasal Inventory-12

The ASK Nasal-12 is a site-specific nasal morbidity instrument developed and validated in 2013 by Little and colleagues[29] to evaluate rhinological PROs following endonasal skull base surgery. An initial 23-item list was created based on expert opinion, review of the literature, and a self-administered survey of patients within 2 weeks preoperatively and at the first postoperative clinic follow-up to assess common rhinological complaints. The initial list was reduced into a final 12-item questionnaire by evaluating the importance and relevance of each item. Each item ranges from "No Problem" to "Severe Problem" on a Likert scale. Patients undergoing endonasal transsphenoidal approach in 3 centers were prospectively enrolled, totaling 104 patients with preoperative questionnaires, of which 100 patients (96%) filled postoperative questionnaires 2 to 4 weeks after surgery, gauging crusting, pain, and ease of breathing. The authors concluded that the ASK Nasal-12 is a site-specific, unidimensional rhinological PRO tool sensitive to clinical change. It can be reliably used to assess nasal PROs in endonasal skull base surgery.

This instrument was used by the same team in 2015 in a prospective cohort multicentric study to compare microscopic and endoscopic transsphenoidal surgery for pituitary adenomas. A total of 218 patients were analyzed and the ASK Nasal 12 assessments were completed before surgery, and 2 weeks, 3 months, and 6 months after surgery. No significant difference was noted between the 2 techniques, both having worse PROs at 2 weeks postop, which returned to baseline at 3 and 6 months after surgery.[40]

Van der Meulen and colleagues[41] used this instrument in a prospective cohort study published in 2022 to assess the influence of patient-reported nasal symptoms on QoL after endoscopic pituitary surgery. Their study included 103 patients undergoing endoscopic pituitary adenoma resection. Nasal symptoms were captured using the ASK Nasal-12 preoperatively, at 5 days, 6 weeks, and 6 months after surgery. Health-related QoL was measured with the Short Form-36 and physical and mental component scores. They identified a significant association between nasal symptoms, particularly olfactory and gustatory problems, and a decrease in physical health-related QoL. The authors concluded that close monitoring of these symptoms may help in optimizing health-related QoL in patients undergoing endoscopic transsphenoidal resection of a pituitary adenoma.

The Suprasellar Meningioma Patient-Reported Outcome Survey

The Suprasellar Meningioma Patient-Reported Outcome Survey (SMPRO) is a disease-specific PROM. It is the first PROM aimed to evaluate the PROs of suprasellar meningioma surgery.[42] Described by Khalafallah and colleagues in 2021, the SMPRO is a 25-item questionnaire, including 17 meningioma specific items combined with 8 items chosen from the Patient-Reported Outcomes Measurement Information System-29 (PROMIS-29). The items were chosen by scoring the relevance of each of the items of the 55-item original list and the 29-item PROMIS-29 using a 1-to-5 Likert scale. Scoring was performed by 15 surgeons and 32 patients. The SMPRO items are split into 9 domains that differ during 3 timepoints: right before surgery, 2 weeks after surgery, and 3 months after surgery.

The final 25-item SMPRO questionnaire was used to compare PROs between patients who underwent a transcranial approach versus endoscopic endonasal approach for resection of a suprasellar meningioma. There was no difference in tumor size, and there was a nonstatistically significative difference in surgery for a recurrent tumor between the 2 groups. Patients who underwent a transcranial approach reported a significantly worse future prospect before surgery, tiredness from medication 2 weeks after surgery, and memory and word-finding difficulties 3 months after surgery. It was also noted that surgeons overestimated their patient's concerns about certain items, especially for blurry vision (preoperatively and postoperatively) and taste issues in the postoperative period. Patients were significantly less concerned about those specific items than their surgeons estimated they would be. The authors concluded that the SMPRO is a disease-specific and approach-specific tool that is reliable in comparing QoL of patients by surgical approach.

The Endoscopic Endonasal Sinus and Skull Base Surgery Questionnaire

The Endoscopic Endonasal Sinus and Skull Base Surgery Questionnaire (EES-Q) was developed to capture the influence of surgery on social QoL and activity, in addition to the physical and psychological reported outcomes. It was created by Ten Dam and colleagues[43] with a 30-item questionnaire, performed on a total of 300 patients, including 93 patients with anterior skull base pathologic condition with the remaining patients having sinus pathologic condition. It was validated at a later stage in a prospective cohort study by confirming significant positive and negative correlations with the SNOT-22. The authors noted that when surgery has a bigger negative social influence on the patient, lower postoperative outcomes were reported.[44] This test adds an interesting perspective to the PROs by collecting the social PROs (impact on work/studying, daily activities, leisure time activities, hobbies, and other social activities) for a better understanding of the needs of the patients, an important step toward offering patients more optimal individualized care. Future validation in a pure skull base surgery population would enhance its value for evaluating PROs in these patients. See **Table 1** for an overview of the PROMs commonly used in patients undergoing endonasal endoscopic skull base surgery.

Overview and Future Directions

Due to the availability of multiple previously developed PROMs applicable in endoscopic skull base surgery cases, it is important to understand the limitations and advantages of each tool. The SNOT-22 was initially developed for the context of endonasal surgery for chronic sinusitis. This proved to be a limitation for assessing patients' QoL after endoscopic pituitary surgery as half of the items did not change from before to after the surgery.[31] This is typical of PROMs used to assess QoL of patient populations for which they were not validated. The SNOT-NC partially addresses this problem by being more neurosurgically oriented. However, as a recent tool, it has not been assessed for test–retest reliability and is only available in German.[36] The ASBQ and SBI are both specific to skull base surgery and were shown to be strongly correlated.[39] However, they are significantly longer than the SNOT-12/NC, with 35 and 41 items each, which may influence rates of patient completion.[45] ASK Nasal-12 is short (12 items) and validated for endoscopic endonasal skull base surgery; however, it is specific for rhinonasal outcomes and does not include other possible postoperative complaints.[29] The SMPRO is another relatively short PROM (25 items) that is validated in endoscopic endonasal and transcranial approaches. However, this PROM was developed specifically for patients with suprasellar meningiomas. Although this may not necessarily be a limitation, some suprasellar meningioma-specific outcomes

Table 1
Overview of patient-reported outcome measurements commonly used in patients undergoing endonasal endoscopic skull base surgery

Patient-Reported Outcomes Measure	Number of Items	Used In	Number of Available Validated Translations	Time Needed to Complete (minutes)
The 22-Item Sino-Nasal Outcome Test	22	Chronic sinusitis[24] Endoscopic endonasal skull base surgery[25–28,31]	13	2–3
The Sino-Nasal Outcome Test for Neurosurgery	23	Endoscopic endonasal skull base surgery[36]	1 (German)	2–3
The Anterior Skull Base Questionnaire	35	Anterior skull base tumors[30]	3	4–5
The Skull Base Inventory	41	Anterior and central skull base pathologic condition[37–39]	1	6–7
The Anterior Skull Base Nasal Inventory-12	12	Endoscopic endonasal skull base surgery[29]	1	1–2
The Sprasellar Meningioma Patient-Reported Outcome Survey	25	Suprasellar meningioma surgery[42]	1	2–3
The Endoscopic Endonasal Sinus and Skull Base Surgery Questionnaire	30	Anterior skull base pathologic condition[43] Sinus pathologic conditions[43]	1	3–4

may not be of relevance in other suprasellar and skull base pathologic conditions.[42] Finally, the EES-Q adds social PROs into its items, which sets it apart from the previously mentioned PROMs. However, it has not yet been validated in a pure skull base surgery population.[43]

Collaboration between neurosurgeons and Ear, Nose, and Throat (ENT) surgeons has been a sought-after trend in endoscopic endonasal skull base surgery. Noh and colleagues[46] compared olfactory and sinonasal outcomes in endoscopic pituitary surgery between patients whose surgery was performed by a single neurosurgeon versus patients who underwent surgery by a collaborative team. Even though they found no difference in the SNOT-22 between the 2 groups, a significative difference was noted in objective olfactory functions using the CC-SIT and BTT scores 3 months after surgery. Better olfaction scores were observed in patients who had surgery with both a neurosurgeon and an ENT surgeon (8.44 ± 3.00 vs 9.84 ± 1.40; $P = .012$ and 4.67 ± 0.84 vs 5.02 ± 0.33; $P = .022$, respectively). This highlights the importance of the collaboration between ENT and neurosurgery teams in endoscopic anterior skull base surgery.

Endoscopic endonasal transsphenoidal surgery may affect olfaction whatever the approach selected, or the precautions taken. Importantly, loss of olfaction can be reversible with time, with younger patients typically having better outcomes.[47] It is important to prepare patients for this eventuality, which helps cushion the influence on QoL.

SUMMARY

PROs are important in assessing the influence of endoscopic endonasal skull base surgery on patients beyond the routinely measured clinical and radiographic data.

This field is currently a subject of extensive research. Digital integration of PROMs into the clinical settings has resulted in improvements in PRO evaluation and patient participation.[48] Advances in this field will undeniably benefit patients and clinicians alike, with patients having access to more personalized approaches to their disease and treatment. Nevertheless, skull base tumors are heterogenous. Many variables including tumor location and size, involvement of vascular structures, hormonal impact, and tumor biology can influence outcomes. Establishing and standardizing PRO collection during the perioperative and follow-up periods can help create a personalized approach to better treat each patient undergoing endoscopic endonasal skull base surgery. This would provide a deeper understanding of the overall influence of surgical nuances on patients by creating better tools adapted to this population.

CLINICS CARE POINTS

- PROs provide insight into what matters most to patients and empowers a patient centered approach.
- Digital integration has resulted in improved access and participation in PROMs.
- Research on PROs for skull base tumors are in its infancy; in the future we will have robust data to enable more informed clinical decisions.

ACKNOWLEDGMENTS

NIH/NCI Cancer Center Support, Grant/Award Number: P30 CA008748.

REFERENCES

1. Moussazadeh N, Prabhu V, Bander ED, et al. Endoscopic endonasal versus open transcranial resection of craniopharyngiomas: a case-matched single-institution analysis. Neurosurg Focus 2016;41(6):E7.
2. Abergel A, Cavel O, Margalit N, et al. Comparison of quality of life after transnasal endoscopic vs open skull base tumor resection. Arch Otolaryngol Head Neck Surg 2012;138(2):142–7.
3. Miller JD, Taylor RJ, Ambrose EC, et al. Complications of open approaches to the skull base in the endoscopic era. J Neurol Surg B Skull Base 2017;78(1):11–7.
4. Brotman JJ, Kotloff RM. Providing outpatient telehealth services in the united states: before and during coronavirus disease 2019. Chest 2021;159(4):1548–58.
5. Guyatt G, Walter S, Norman G. Measuring change over time: assessing the usefulness of evaluative instruments. J Chronic Dis 1987;40(2):171–8.
6. Cella D, Hahn EA, Dineen K. Meaningful change in cancer-specific quality of life scores: differences between improvement and worsening. Qual Life Res 2002; 11(3):207–21.
7. Maringwa J, Quinten C, King M, et al. Minimal clinically meaningful differences for the EORTC QLQ-C30 and EORTC QLQ-BN20 scales in brain cancer patients. Ann Oncol 2011;22(9):2107–12.
8. Amit M, Abergel A, Fliss DM, et al. The clinical importance of quality-of-life scores in patients with skull base tumors: a meta-analysis and review of the literature. Head Neck Cancers 2012;14:175–81.
9. Croy I, Nordin S, Hummel T. Olfactory disorders and quality of life–an updated review. Chem senses 2014;39(3):185–94.

10. Majovsky M, Astl J, Kovar D, et al. Olfactory function in patients after transsphenoidal surgery for pituitary adenomas-a short review. Neurosurg Rev 2019;42(2): 395–401.
11. Landis BN, Hummel T, Hugentobler M, et al. Ratings of overall olfactory function. Chem Senses 2003;28(8):691–4.
12. Kahilogullari G, Beton S, Al-Beyati ESM, et al. Olfactory functions after transsphenoidal pituitary surgery: endoscopic versus microscopic approach. Laryngoscope 2013;123(9):2112–9.
13. Hadad G, Bassagasteguy L, Carrau RL, et al. A novel reconstructive technique after endoscopic expanded endonasal approaches: vascular pedicle nasoseptal flap. Laryngoscope 2006;116(10):1882–6.
14. Rivera-Serrano CM, Snyderman CH, Gardner P, et al. Nasoseptal "rescue" flap: a novel modification of the nasoseptal flap technique for pituitary surgery. Laryngoscope 2011;121(5):990–3.
15. Tam S, Duggal N, Rotenberg BW. Olfactory outcomes following endoscopic pituitary surgery with or without septal flap reconstruction: a randomized controlled trial. Int Forum Allergy Rhinol 2013;3(1):62–5.
16. Doty RL, Shaman P, Kimmelman CP, et al. University of Pennsylvania Smell Identification Test: a rapid quantitative olfactory function test for the clinic. Laryngoscope 1984;94(2 Pt 1):176–8.
17. Puccinelli CL, Yin LX, O'Brien EK, et al. Long-term olfaction outcomes in transnasal endoscopic skull-base surgery: a prospective cohort study comparing electrocautery and cold knife upper septal limb incision techniques. Int Forum Allergy Rhinol 2019;9(5):493–500.
18. Doty RL, Marcus A, William Lee W. Development of the 12-item Cross-Cultural Smell Identification Test (CC-SIT). Laryngoscope 1996;106(3 Pt 1):353–6.
19. Kobal G, Hummel T, Sekinger B, et al. "Sniffin" sticks": screening of olfactory performance. Rhinology 1996;34(4):222–6. Available at: https://europepmc.org/article/med/9050101. Accessed January 16, 2022.
20. Pusswald G, Auff E, Lehrner J. Development of a brief self-report inventory to measure olfactory dysfunction and quality of life in patients with problems with the sense of smell. Chemosensory Perception 2012;5(3–4):292–9.
21. Cain WS, Gent JF, Goodspeed R, et al. Evaluation of olfactory dysfunction in the connecticut chemosensory clinical research center. Laryngoscope 1988; 98(1):83–8.
22. Raikundalia MD, Huang RJ, Chan L, et al. Olfactory-specific quality of life outcomes after endoscopic endonasal surgery of the sella. Allergy Rhinol (Providence) 2021;12. https://doi.org/10.1177/21526567211045041.
23. Hopkins C, Gillett S, Slack R, et al. Psychometric validity of the 22-item Sinonasal Outcome Test. Clin Otolaryngol 2009;34(5):447–54.
24. Farhood Z, Schlosser RJ, Pearse ME, et al. Twenty-two-item Sino-Nasal Outcome Test in a control population: a cross-sectional study and systematic review. Int Forum Allergy Rhinol 2016;6(3):271–7.
25. Glicksman JT, Parasher AK, Brooks SG, et al. Sinonasal quality of life after endoscopic resection of malignant sinonasal and skull base tumors. Laryngoscope 2018;128(4):789–93.
26. McCoul ED, Anand VK, Bedrosian JC, et al. Endoscopic skull base surgery and its impact on sinonasal-related quality of life. Int Forum Allergy Rhinol 2012;2(2):174–81.
27. Riley CA, Tabaee A, Conley L, et al. Long-term sinonasal outcomes after endoscopic skull base surgery with nasoseptal flap reconstruction. Laryngoscope 2019;129(5):1035–40.

28. Patel KS, Raza SM, McCoul ED, et al. Long-term quality of life after endonasal endoscopic resection of adult craniopharyngiomas. J Neurosurg 2015;123(3):571–80.
29. Little AS, Kelly D, Milligan J, et al. Prospective validation of a patient-reported nasal quality-of-life tool for endonasal skull base surgery: the Anterior Skull Base Nasal Inventory-12. J Neurosurg 2013;119(4):1068–74.
30. Gil Z, Abergel A, Spektor S, et al. Development of a cancer-specific anterior skull base quality-of-life questionnaire. J Neurosurg 2004;100(5):813–9.
31. Sarris CE, Little AS, Kshettry VR, et al. Assessment of the validity of the sinonasal outcomes test-22 in pituitary surgery: a multicenter prospective trial. Laryngoscope 2021;131(11):E2757–63.
32. de Almeida JR, Snyderman CH, Gardner PA, et al. Nasal morbidity following endoscopic skull base surgery: a prospective cohort study. Head Neck 2011;33(4):547–51.
33. Chabot JD, Patel CR, Hughes MA, et al. Nasoseptal flap necrosis: a rare complication of endoscopic endonasal surgery. J Neurosurg 2018;128(5):1463–72.
34. Lavigne P, Faden DL, Wang EW, et al. Complications of nasoseptal flap reconstruction: a systematic review. J Neurol Surg B Skull Base 2018;79(Suppl 4):S291–9.
35. Bhenswala PN, Schlosser RJ, Nguyen SA, et al. Sinonasal quality-of-life outcomes after endoscopic endonasal skull base surgery. Int Forum Allergy Rhinol 2019;9(10):1105–18.
36. Ahmadipour Y, Müller O, Kreitschmann-Andermahr I, et al. Development, reliability, validity and sensitivity of the Sino-Nasal Outcome Test for Neurosurgery (SNOT-NC). Eur Arch Otorhinolaryngol 2020;277(1):235–44.
37. de Almeida JR, Vescan AD, Gullane PJ, et al. Development of a disease-specific quality-of-life questionnaire for anterior and central skull base pathology–the skull base inventory. Laryngoscope 2012;122(9):1933–42.
38. Larjani S, Monteiro E, Witterick I, et al. Preliminary cross-sectional reliability and validity of the Skull Base Inventory (SBI) quality of life questionnaire. J Otolaryngol Head Neck Surg 2016. https://doi.org/10.1186/s40463-016-0158-y.
39. Forner D, Hueniken K, Yoannidis T, et al. Psychometric testing of the Skull Base Inventory health-related quality of life questionnaire in a multi-institutional study of patients undergoing open and endoscopic surgery. Qual Life Res 2021;30:293–301.
40. Little AS, Kelly DF, Milligan J, et al. Comparison of sinonasal quality of life and health status in patients undergoing microscopic and endoscopic transsphenoidal surgery for pituitary lesions: a prospective cohort study. J Neurosurg 2015;123(3):799–807.
41. van der Meulen M, Verstegen MJT, Lobatto DJ, et al. Impact of patient-reported nasal symptoms on quality of life after endoscopic pituitary surgery: a prospective cohort study. Pituitary 2022. https://doi.org/10.1007/S11102-021-01199-4.
42. Khalafallah AM, Rakovec M, Burapachaisri K, et al. The suprasellar meningioma patient-reported outcome survey: a disease-specific patient-reported outcome measure for resection of suprasellar meningioma. J Neurosurg 2021;1(aop):1–9.
43. ten Dam E, Feijen RA, van den Berge MJC, et al. Development of the Endoscopic Endonasal Sinus and Skull Base Surgery Questionnaire. Int Forum Allergy Rhinol 2017;7(11):1076–84.
44. ten Dam E, Korsten-Meijer AGW, Hoving EW, et al. Evaluation of the psychometric properties of the endoscopic endonasal sinus and skull base surgery questionnaire (EES-Q) in a prospective cohort study. Clin Otolaryngol 2019;44(4):565–71.

45. Edwards P, Roberts I, Clarke M, et al. Increasing response rates to postal questionnaires: systematic review. BMJ 2002;324(7347):1183–5.
46. Noh Y, Choi JE, Lee KE, et al. A comparison of olfactory and sinonasal outcomes in endoscopic pituitary surgery performed by a single neurosurgeon or a collaborative team of surgeons. Clin Exp Otorhinolaryngol 2020;13(3):261–7.
47. Kim BY, Kang SG, Kim SW, et al. Olfactory changes after endoscopic endonasal transsphenoidal approach for skull base tumors. Laryngoscope 2014;124(11):2470–5.
48. Lavallee DC, Chenok KE, Love RM, et al. Incorporating patient-reported outcomes into health care to engage patients and enhance care. Health Aff (Millwood) 2017;35(4):575–82.

Quality of Life in Patients with Adrenal Insufficiency

Dingfeng Li, MD, MSc*

KEYWORDS

• Cortisol • Disease burden • Self-perceived health • Health-care delivery

KEY POINTS

- Patients with adrenal insufficiency continue to experience impaired self-perceived health status and quality of life despite glucocorticoid replacement therapy.
- Patients with different subtypes of adrenal insufficiency all suffer from impaired quality of life, more profound in secondary adrenal insufficiency and glucocorticoid-induced adrenal insufficiency, when compared with general population.
- Factors that are associated with quality of life include patient's age, gender, duration and types of adrenal insufficiency, steroid replacement strategy, insurance coverage, financial burden from adrenal insufficiency, and family support.
- Clinicians should emphasize modifiable factors to improve patients' quality of life.
- The coronavirus disease pandemic has posed new challenges on patient's quality of life. Awareness and action are needed from treating clinicians.

INTRODUCTION

Adrenal Insufficiency and Its Main Subtypes

Adrenal insufficiency is a common chronic endocrine condition characterized by glucocorticoid deficiency with or without concomitant mineralocorticoid deficiency.[1] By the underlying cause, it can be further categorized into 2 main subtypes: primary adrenal insufficiency (PAI) and secondary adrenal insufficiency (SAI). PAI is caused by intrinsic disease of the adrenal glands, whereas SAI is due to disorders affecting the pituitary gland or the hypothalamus that lead to impaired secretion of adrenocorticotropic hormone.[1] As a very common but unique subtype, glucocorticoid-induced adrenal insufficiency (GIAI) is frequently encountered in both endocrinology and non-endocrinology practices. It is secondary to chronic high-dose glucocorticoid usage, which leads to suppression of the hypothalamus-pituitary-adrenal axis.[2] It has been controversial whether GIAI should be categorized as tertiary adrenal insufficiency vs SAI. In this review, we will discuss GIAI separate from SAI, due to its unique pathophysiology and challenges in management.[2]

Department of Endocrinology, Endocrine and Metabolism Institute, Cleveland Clinic, 9500 Euclid Avenue, F20, Cleveland, OH 44195, USA
* Corresponding author.
E-mail address: lid12@ccf.org

Endocrinol Metab Clin N Am 51 (2022) 741–753
https://doi.org/10.1016/j.ecl.2022.04.003

Quality of Life Questionnaires for Adrenal Insufficiency

Quantitative assessments of quality of life involves administration of questionnaires. Depending on the target disease and/or patient population, there are 2 types of questionnaires: (1) general questionnaires that evaluate dimensions common to a wide variety of conditions or healthy population and (2) disease-specific questionnaires that focus on a particular group of patients with the disease of interest.[3] In patients with adrenal insufficiency, the most commonly used questionnaires are Short Form-36 (a general questionnaire), and Addison's Quality of Life Questionnaire (AddiQoL) (a disease-specific questionnaire).

General questionnaire: Short Form-36

The Short Form-36 has been widely used in numerous outcome studies in the medical literature. It is a patient self-assessment including 8 dimensions of quality of life during the preceding 4 weeks. These dimensions are physical functioning, role-physical limitation, bodily pain, general health, vitality, social functioning, role-emotional limitation, and mental health.[4] In each dimension, the range is 0 to 100, with higher scores indicating less pain, better functioning, or performance.[5] Four dimensions (physical functioning, role-physical limitation, bodily pain, and general health) may be merged into a comprehensive index for physical functioning (the physical component summary), whereas the other 4 dimensions (vitality, social functioning, role-emotional limitation, and mental health) may compose a comprehensive index of mental functioning (the mental component summary), using a prespecified formula.[6,7] Mean score and standard deviation by age/decade and sex of the general population in each individual country are published and available to be served as referent values.[8] Although developed as a general questionnaire, Short Form-36 has been widely used as a quantitative metric of quality of life in patients with adrenal insufficiency by multiple studies and clinical trials.[9–13]

Disease-specific health-related questionnaire: AddiQoL

A disease-specific quality of life questionnaire for patients with Addison disease, AddiQoL, was initially developed and pretested as a preliminary questionnaire in 100 patients with Addison disease from the UK Addison's Disease Self-Help Group in 2010.[14] It was subsequently modified, finalized, and validated in 2012 at 5 European centers.[15] The final questionnaires can be administered as a full version that contains 30 items (AddiQoL-30), or as a short version that contains 8 items focusing exclusively on fatigue (AddiQoL-8). The AddiQoL-30 assesses 4 dimensions: fatigue (8 items), emotions (8 items), symptoms (9 items), and miscellaneous (sleep, sexuality, and impact of intercurrent disease, 5 items). A score range of 1 to 4 is given to each item. A higher score indicates a higher level of quality of life, with a maximum score of 120. AddiQoL-30 has high reliability with Cronbach α-coefficient 0.93 and Person separation index 0.86, as well as good correlation with Short Form-36.[14] AddiQoL-8 also proved valid and reliable.[15] Although developed and validated in patients with Addison disease within the European Network, because symptomatology overlaps and exists in all subtypes of adrenal insufficiency, AddiQoL has been extrapolated to patients with SAI in multiple subsequent quality of life studies, as well as in other countries and populations.[16–20]

QUALITY OF LIFE BY SUBTYPE OF ADRENAL INSUFFICIENCY

Quality of life in primary adrenal insufficiency

Quality of life in patients with PAI was first systematically described in 79 Norwegian patients by Lovas and colleagues in 2002.[21] This study used Short Form-36 and Fatigue questionnaires and compared patients with PAI to general population in Norway.

The authors demonstrated that the general health and vitality perception were most consistently impaired in these patients among the 8 dimensions of Short Form-36, and that patients with solitary PAI had better quality of life than those with PAI plus concomitant autoimmune conditions.[21] Similar findings were reported by another 2 studies, with a larger number of patients with PAI.[22,23] However, these 3 studies were limited by only including patients with autoimmune PAI (Addison disease), whereas data regarding other causes of PAI, as well as comparison to patients with SAI, remained unknown. Several subsequent cross-sectional survey studies in Europe were conducted to fill this gap. In a study by Hahner and colleagues in 2007, 131 patients with PAI, that included all causes of PAI, were found to have lower scores in 7 of the 8 domains of Short Form-36 (with the exception of body pain) compared with 660 matched controls who did not have adrenal insufficiency.[24] Using 2 other questionnaires, the Giessen Complaint List and Hospital Anxiety and Depression Scale (HADS), they also found a lower score in general subjective health status and higher level of anxiety. It was postulated that this might be multifactorial: from other concomitant autoimmune disorders, concurrent mineralocorticoid deficiency, and vulnerability to adrenal crisis.[24] These differences remained significant even after exclusion of all patients with concomitant diseases as a confounding factor.[24] Two recent US studies concurred with the findings that patients with PAI experienced the highest frequency of adrenal crises compared with other adrenal insufficiency subtypes, and these patients reported impaired quality of life compared with the age/sex-matched general population.[13,25] From a socioeconomical level, reduced health-related quality of life is associated with reduced employability, as proven by a high proportion of patients with PAI on sickness pensions,[22] which might also associate with worsened quality of life.

Quality of life in secondary adrenal insufficiency

Patients with SAI have also been shown to have impaired quality of life compared with general population. Patients with a history of pituitary disease, such as Cushing disease, acromegaly, and craniopharyngioma, were historically reported to experience a long-term impaired quality of life after structurally or biochemically curative surgeries.[26–29] However, these studies individually focused on a specific pituitary disease and whether these patients developed SAI following the surgery were not consistently confirmed. The seminal study that reported quality of life in patients with SAI is the aforementioned article by Hahner and colleagues in 2007.[24] In this study, 78 patients with SAI due to pituitary disease reported lower scores in 7 of the 8 domains of Short Form-36 (except for body pain) compared with 660 matched controls who did not have adrenal insufficiency.[24] The authors also found that SAI patients were slightly more compromised than patients with PAI, especially in two Short Form-36 dimensions (physical functioning and body pain) and the HADS depression score, whereas other dimensions of Short Form-36 were not significantly different, possibly due to smaller sample size and insufficient power.[24] Similar findings were replicated and reported in several subsequent European studies by Bleicken and colleagues,[9–11] as well as in 2 recent US studies.[13,25] It suggested that concomitant endocrine disease and other pituitary hormonal deficiencies, which are common in the context of SAI due to hypopituitarism, may contribute to impaired subjective health status.[24,27,30,31] In addition to these factors, patient's self-report of a higher level of discomfort with self-management, lower compliance rate with wearing medical alert gear or having injectable glucocorticoid at home, and higher likelihood of delays in the emergency department when having adrenal crisis in patients with SAI than those with PAI, could all play a role and explain the differences, which also reflected a gap in current management and patient education.[13,25]

Quality of life in glucocorticoid induced adrenal insufficiency

Although GIAI is believed to be the most common cause of adrenal insufficiency and is frequently encountered in clinical practice, the true prevalence is unclear and it represents a vastly heterogeneous population with various underlying primary causes.[2] To date, very few studies have evaluated quality of life in this patient group separately from the other 2 subtypes. A US study at 2 tertiary centers in 2020, which did not assess quality of life with a systematical questionnaire, reported that patients with GIAI had the highest proportion of subjective feelings of poor health in general, compared with those with PAI and SAI.[25] A subsequent study using Short Form-36 questionnaires in a broader network and larger sample size (N = 529), demonstrated a significantly lower quality of life in patients with GIAI, especially within the physical component summary score, which was 25% lower than in patients with PAI and SAI.[13] These patients also experienced highest number of adrenal crises per person-year compared with PAI and SAI. Notably, patients with GIAI had the lowest availability of injectable glucocorticoids, the lowest compliance with wearing medical alert gear, and reported the highest self-perceived difficulty with self-management of adrenal insufficiency.[13] These findings reflected a substantial gap in risk recognition, patient and caregiver counseling and education, also reported in several other studies.[32–34] As a limitation, the authors acknowledged that patients with GIAI may often have an underlying inflammatory condition that may independently contribute to impaired quality of life, which was not captured or described by the questionnaires.[13,35] Another recent survey study by Mehta and colleagues, based on rheumatology practice in the United Kingdom concurred with these findings. It reported that 26% of patients with GIAI were never evaluated by endocrinologists, that 50% of rheumatology providers did not routinely counsel patients on the sick day rules, and that only 13% of rheumatologists followed the recent adrenal insufficiency treatment guidelines.[36] These studies suggest there is unmet need and gap existing in current practice in this group of patients, who warrants more attention in the diagnosis and treatment of adrenal insufficiency.

DETERMINANTS OF QUALITY OF LIFE

Patient's gender and age

Lovas and colleagues reported that female patients with PAI (Addison's disease only) had lower scores in 2 Short Form-36 dimensions—physical functioning and role-emotional limitation.[21] Lower quality of life in female patients with PAI or SAI, was also observed in another subsequent study by Hahner and colleagues, in vitality and mental health. However, in this study, after adjusting the scores with normative scores from the referent population, they were similar between men and women.[24] In a more recent study with a larger cohort of 529 patients of PAI, SAI, or GIAI, from three centers in the United States, after multivariate adjustment, female sex was associated with a lower age/sex adjusted score in both physical component summary and mental component summary of Short Form-36.[13] These data, although not always consistent, suggest women with adrenal insufficiency could be more vulnerable than men, and may warrant more attention from treating clinicians. With regard to patient's age, one European study reported that older age was associated with lower score in body pain and with higher score in general health,[24] whereas another American study found no difference between current age and quality of life.[13] The discrepant findings may be due to differences in ethnicity, cultural or religious background, and whether potential confounding factors being accounted for. From this perspective, future larger studies that include a more diverse patient population are needed.

Subtype and duration of adrenal insufficiency

Although overall, patients with adrenal insufficiency reported more impaired quality of life when compared with the general population, studies that compared patients with different subtypes of adrenal insufficiency demonstrated differences of quality of life.[12,13,24,25] Notably, patients with PAI reported relatively higher quality of life scores than those with SAI due to pituitary diseases,[12,13,24,25] and those with adrenal insufficiency due to iatrogenic glucocorticoid usage.[12,13,25] Several factors could explain why patients with PAI had better self-perceived health status and quality of life, for example, absence of other pituitary hormone deficiency, a younger patient population, a longer duration of disease, better education and a higher degree of knowledge of disease in patients, higher compliance with wearing medical alert gear, higher availability of injectable glucocorticoid, a higher comfort level with self-management, and a better support system.[24,25] Based on two studies with multivariable analysis from a large cohorts of patients, after adjusting for these factors, patients with PAI were still two-fold more likely to report better subjective health status and quality of life, especially in the physical component summary, compared with other subtypes.[13,25] Regarding the duration of adrenal insufficiency, limited data exist with one study reporting no impact of duration on quality of life,[24] whereas another study demonstrating that patients with shorter duration (less than 6 years from time of diagnosis to the time of survey) were more likely to report a lower score in physical and mental component summary of Short Form-36.[25]

Glucocorticoid replacement

Impaired quality of life in patients with adrenal insufficiency occurs despite standard glucocorticoid replacement therapy. Whether the selection of glucocorticoid formulation, dosage, frequency, and route of administration has impact on quality of life has been a research interest. Oral hydrocortisone in 2 to 3 divided dosages is the most common, and conventional formulation of glucocorticoid replacement regimen, although other oral regimens such as cortisone acetate, prednisone, prednisolone, and rarely dexamethasone can be used in clinical practice depending on clinical scenarios.[1] To date, there is only one study by Bleicken and colleagues in 2008, which compared different glucocorticoid formulations, that demonstrated patients taking hydrocortisone or cortisone acetate had better quality of life than those taking prednisolone in the body pain dimension.[9] However, overall the author concluded that prednisolone seemed to be equivalent to other formulations regarding subjective health status in patients with adrenal insufficiency.[9]

Modified release hydrocortisone formulations such as Plenadren and Chronocort are novel glucocorticoid replacement therapies aiming to replicate the circadian rhythm more closely than conventional hydrocortisone. Plenadren is a dual-release preparation of hydrocortisone administered orally once daily,[37] approved and available in Europe. In an open prospective trial of 50 patients with PAI or SAI taking conventional hydrocortisone therapy, 30 patients switched to Plenadren. Quality of life scores by AddiQoL were similar after the switch, whereas there was a significant decrease in scores in those patients who remained on conventional therapy.[16] Another study of 19 patients with PAI due to Addison disease showed significant improvement in AddiQoL scores 12 months after switching from conventional hydrocortisone to

Plenadren.[38] In a recent larger single-blinded randomized controlled trial of 89 patients with PAI or SAI, improvement in AddiQoL scores was also reported at 24 weeks following initiation of Plenadren.[19] However, in a prospective, open-label, multicenter, 5-year extension study, quality of life scores remained unchanged from baseline to 5 years.[20] Chronocort is another new modified release hydrocortisone that is still under development.[39] Although studies have shown it has better androgen control, with increased lean body mass and bone formation marker compared with conventional therapy,[39–41] however, to date, its impact on patient's quality of life has not been reported.

Continuous subcutaneous hydrocortisone infusion is an emerging therapeutic option, primarily in patients with PAI due to classic congenital adrenal hyperplasia, or Addison disease. Due to the rarity of the diseases, data exist from case reports and small-scale randomized clinical trials and are not very consistent.[42–46] Despite a more circadian pattern of cortisol release, some studies did not observe improved quality of life with subcutaneous hydrocortisone infusion, casting doubt on the potential quality of life effects of circadian cortisol delivery.[42,46] Several other studies showed that long-term use of continuous subcutaneous hydrocortisone infusion seemed to be a safe and well-tolerated treatment option and improved subjective health status in a selected set of patients, especially in those poorly controlled on conventional therapy who suffered from a lower baseline quality of life.[43–45] It should be noted that continuous subcutaneous hydrocortisone infusion is not the standard-of-care treatment and is not available to most patients with adrenal insufficiency in most countries.

Regarding the impact of glucocorticoid dosage on quality of life, Hahner's study in 2007 reported that a higher dose of glucocorticoid was associated with higher physical functioning score and lower physical role limitation score.[24] A subsequent study from a similar network of patients in 2010 found that patients on doses greater than 30 mg/d hydrocortisone showed a significantly impaired quality of life especially for physical role limitation score and general health score, when compared with sex-matched and age-matched controls. In addition, patients on hydrocortisone with thrice daily intake showed significantly impaired quality of life in social functioning (15–20 mg/d, 20–25 mg/d).[10] A randomized controlled trial in Netherlands demonstrated that patients receiving higher doses of hydrocortisone (0.4–0.6 mg/kg body weight/d) reported less general and mental fatigue, better overall health, and more vitality.[47] However, another randomized, double-blind study showed no difference in cognition, memory, attention, or executive function when patients were treated with a higher dose of hydrocortisone (30–40 mg daily).[48] One study in the United States reported self-perceived poor health was associated with taking higher doses of glucocorticoid (>25 mg/d hydrocortisone equivalence).[25] Another recent study from 3 centers in the United States, demonstrated that taking daily dosage greater than 25 mg hydrocortisone equivalence was associated with a more impaired quality of life especially in the physical component summary of Short Form-36, compared with their sex/decade-matched general population.[13] Therefore, it is prudent for clinician to carefully adjust the dosage to achieve a balance between minimizing underreplacement symptoms and avoiding supraphysiologic dosage during regular follow-up and communication between patients and providers.[25,49]

Mineralocorticoid replacement

Although mineralocorticoid replacement is primarily indicated in patients with PAI, there is small proportion of patients with SAI and GIAI who also take mineralocorticoid on a daily basis.[25] To date, there is no study that has systematically evaluated the association between mineralocorticoid replacement and patient's quality of life.

Dehydroepiandrosterone replacement

Both PAI and SAI results in long-term low or undetectable regarding dehydroepiandrosterone (DHEA) levels.[50] To date, there have been several clinical trials investigating its utility in female patients with adrenal insufficiency, and data in men are still lacking. The first randomized, double-blind, placebo-controlled trial was conducted in 24 women with PAI or SAI by Arlt and colleagues, which observed improved overall well-being and depression and anxiety scores with DHEA replacement.[51] Several subsequent small-scale studies were conducted with various reports and inconclusive results regarding DHEA replacement on psychological function, mood, cognition, sexual functions, lean body mass, and bone density.[52,53] A meta-analysis of 10 studies of DHEA replacement in women with PAI and SAI showed subtle improvement in the quality of life and depression symptoms; no change in libido or anxiety was observed with DHEA replacement.[54] Therapeutic regimens in clinical trials have usually given DHEA administered in physiologic doses of 25 to 50 mg/d.[51–53] However, DHEA is widely available over the counter as supplements in the United States or via Internet commercials without FDA oversight for potency or duration of action. Quality control of DHEA has been shown to be inconsistent,[55] which could lead to various response in quality of life. Overreplacement could lead to androgenic side effects (acne and hirsutism), which are of concern for long-term administration.[56] In conclusion, there is insufficient evidence to support routine use of DHEA in women with adrenal insufficiency. The initiation of treatment could be considered in a subset of women with severe androgen deficiency on a case-by-case basis through shared decision-making with appropriate subsequent monitoring.[1]

Socioeconomic factors

Patients with adrenal insufficiency may also experience adversities related to socioeconomic level. These factors, including insurance coverage, financial burden from having adrenal insufficiency, and domestic support from family members are not always given sufficient attention in medical practice, despite the fact that they have been identified as important factors that affect quality of life.[25] A retrospective French study demonstrated that adrenal insufficiency was associated with higher rates of unemployment compared with the general population.[57] Another US-based study reported that 16% of patients with adrenal insufficiency reported insufficient coverage from their medical insurance, whereas 44% attributed adrenal insufficiency as the cause of their financial burden, causing inability to work in 10% of patients.[25] Hahner and colleagues also reported that 40% of all patients with adrenal insufficiency had occupational changes due to their adrenal diseases with a total of 18% being out of work and receiving disability pensions, compared with 4% of the general German population around a similar time.[24] In a more recent study, patients with adrenal insufficiency who report higher self-perceived difficulty with self-management were more than 2-fold more likely to report a lower physical component summary score and mental component summary score of Short Form-36.[13] Those patient who lacked a good domestic support system were 9-fold more likely to have a lower mental component summary score.[13] These data underscore the importance of ensuring good insurance coverage to reduce patient financial burden, and more robust hands-on education programs offered to the patients and their family, to ensure better understanding of the disease and management strategies, which were shown to be associated with a better quality of life.[13,25]

Adrenal crisis

Adrenal crisis is one of the most serious and life-threatening manifestations of adrenal insufficiency due to acute absolute or relative glucocorticoid and mineralocorticoid deficiency.[58] Despite standard replacement, adrenal crisis still occurs, with an estimated incidence rate of 4.1 to 24 per 100 patient years,[25,59–62] and it remains as one of the leading causes of death in this population.[63] Data are limited on how adrenal crisis affects patient's quality of life, although it is thought to be substantial.[58] In the recent study by Li and colleagues, patients who had experienced at least one adrenal crisis since their diagnosis of adrenal insufficiency were 2-fold more likely to report impaired self-perceived health status, even after adjusting for age, sex, and type of adrenal insufficiency.[25] This study also demonstrated that patients with adrenal insufficiency, especially those with SAI and GIAI, encountered significant delays in proper treatment of adrenal crisis in the emergency department, and they often thought they were not understood by health-care professionals when explaining adrenal crisis.[25] Whether these factors all contribute to quality of life impairment remains unclear and could be a future research direction.

It should be noted that among the factors listed above, certain factors such as demographics (ie, gender, age, duration, and subtypes of adrenal insufficiency) are nonmodifiable, whereas others, including steroid replacement, socioeconomic factors, as well as vigilance, prevention and timely treatment of adrenal crisis, are modifiable and achievable. Clinicians should be aware of these factors, and strive to optimize patients' quality of life from these perspectives.

IMPACT OF CORONAVIRUS DISEASE ON QUALITY OF LIFE IN PATIENTS WITH ADRENAL INSUFFICIENCY

Since March 2020, the coronavirus disease (COVID-19) pandemic has caused significant impact on our society, economy, and health care and has remained as a public health threat despite mandated vaccinations and the development of new drugs.[64] It has also posed a new challenge in the management of adrenal insufficiency as patients with adrenal insufficiency were thought to be susceptible to infections due to their inefficient innate immune system[65] and are prone to developing adrenal crises from insufficient hypothalamus–pituitary–adrenal axis activation in response to stressors.[19] Although several professional medical societies published expert opinion on how to manage adrenal insufficiency during the pandemic,[66,67] a limited number of original studies have assessed quality of life during the pandemic. One Italian cross-sectional survey study of 121 patients focusing on psychological stress from February 2020 to April 2020 reported patients' concerns on personal health, finances, and quality of life.[17] Patients with PAI and SAI reported similar scores by AddiQoL-30 and Short Form-36 during the pandemic. A negative correlation was found between quality of life and the degree of concern for the pandemic.[17] The only study to date with a direct peripandemic comparison was conducted as part of longitudinal cohort of 342 patients, from 2 large tertiary referral networks in the United States.[12] This study described similar quality of life scores before and after the onset of the pandemic in most dimensions of Short Form-36, with a slightly higher score in the physical component summary score during the pandemic.[12] This study also concluded that about one-third of patients with adrenal insufficiency reported increasing challenges in adrenal insufficiency management during the pandemic, especially younger patients, women, and those experiencing poor access to health care, or with higher financial burden.[12] These challenges with adrenal insufficiency self-management in turn were associated with higher anxiety and stress.[12] Although more studies could still be currently conducted to further assess quality of life in this patient population, these 2 studies are calling for a more robust education, easily accessible health care, and societal support, for patients with adrenal insufficiency to prevent acute events, to reduce psychosocial stress, and to improve quality of life during this still ongoing pandemic.[12,17]

SUMMARY

Patients with adrenal insufficiency are faced with many challenging adversities on multiple levels—patient, clinician, and societal support, which all contribute to impaired subjective health status and quality of life. It is crucial to realize these adversities and the gaps that exist in current practice. Treating clinicians should strive to improve awareness of the disease, to offer comprehensive patient education and counseling, as well as to reduce health-care and financial burdens to this patient population.

CLINICS CARE POINTS

- Patients with adrenal insufficiency continue to report impaired subjective health status and quality of life despite standard glucocorticoid replacement therapy.
- Patients with glucocorticoid-induced adrenal insufficiency report worse quality of life compared with other subtypes, which has not been given sufficient attention or addressed in both endocrine and nonendocrine practices.
- Certain factors associated with quality of life are nonmodifiable (patient's age, gender, duration, and subtypes of adrenal insufficiency), whereas others are modifiable and achievable, including steroid replacement strategy, insurance coverage, financial burden from adrenal insufficiency, patient education, and family support.
- A multidimensional effort is needed to identify patients with high risk of developing adverse outcomes, to ensure adequate patient education, and to offer sufficient support in patients with adrenal insufficiency.
- Coronavirus disease pandemic has posed new challenges on patient's quality of life. Awareness and actions are needed from treating clinicians.

DISCLOSURE

The author has no financial disclosures.

REFERENCES

1. Hahner S, Ross RJ, Arlt W, et al. Adrenal insufficiency. Nat Rev Dis Primers 2021;7(1):19.
2. Prete A, Bancos I. Glucocorticoid induced adrenal insufficiency. BMJ 2021;374:n1380.
3. Ho W, Druce M. Quality of life in patients with adrenal disease: A systematic review. Clin Endocrinol (Oxf) 2018;89(2):119–28.
4. Ware JE Jr, Sherbourne CD. The MOS 36-item short-form health survey (SF-36). I. Conceptual framework and item selection. Med Care 1992;30(6):473–83.

5. Ware JE Jr, Kosinski M, Bayliss MS, McHorney CA, Rogers WH, Raczek A. Comparison of methods for the scoring and statistical analysis of SF-36 health profile and summary measures: summary of results from the medical outcomes study. Med Care 1995;33(4 Suppl):AS264–79.
6. Ware JE, Kosinski M. SF-36 physical & mental health summary scales: a manual for users of version 1. Lincoln, RI: Quality Metric Incorporated; 2001.
7. Taft C, Karlsson J, Sullivan M. Do SF-36 summary component scores accurately summarize subscale scores? Qual Life Res 2001;10(5):395–404.
8. Ware JE, Kosinski M, Turner-Bowker DM, Gandeck B. User's manual for the SF-12v2TM health survey:(with a supplement documenting SF-12 health survey). RI: QualityMetric Incorporated Lincoln; 2007.
9. Bleicken B, Hahner S, Loeffler M, Ventz M, Allolio B, Quinkler M. Impaired subjective health status in chronic adrenal insufficiency: impact of different glucocorticoid replacement regimens. Eur J Endocrinol 2008;159(6):811–7.
10. Bleicken B, Hahner S, Loeffler M, et al. Influence of hydrocortisone dosage scheme on health-related quality of life in patients with adrenal insufficiency. Clin Endocrinol (Oxf) 2010;72(3):297–304.
11. Bleicken B, Hahner S, Ventz M, Quinkler M. Delayed diagnosis of adrenal insufficiency is common: a cross-sectional study in 216 patients. Am J Med Sci 2010; 339(6):525–31.
12. Li D, Suresh M, Abbondanza T, Vaidya A, Bancos I. The impact of the COVID-19 pandemic on self-reported outcomes in patients with adrenal insufficiency. J Clin Endocrinol Metab 2021;106(7):e2469–79.
13. Li D, Brand S, Hamidi O, et al. Quality of life and its determinants in patients with adrenal insufficiency: a survey study at three centers in the USA. J Clin Endocrinol Metab 2022;29. https://doi.org/10.1210/clinem/dgac175.
14. Lovas K, Curran S, Oksnes M, Husebye ES, Huppert FA, Chatterjee VK. Development of a disease-specific quality of life questionnaire in Addison's disease. J Clin Endocrinol Metab 2010;95(2):545–51.
15. Oksnes M, Bensing S, Hulting AL, et al. Quality of life in European patients with Addison's disease: validity of the disease-specific questionnaire AddiQoL. J Clin Endocrinol Metab 2012;97(2):568–76.
16. Quinkler M, Miodini Nilsen R, Zopf K, Ventz M, Oksnes M. Modified-release hydrocortisone decreases BMI and HbA1c in patients with primary and secondary adrenal insufficiency. Eur J Endocrinol 2015;172(5):619–26.
17. Martino M, Aboud N, Cola MF, et al. Impact of COVID-19 pandemic on psychophysical stress in patients with adrenal insufficiency: the CORTI-COVID study. J Endocrinol Invest 2021;44(5):1075–84.
18. Mongioi LM, Condorelli RA, La Vignera S, Calogero AE. Dual-release hydrocortisone treatment: glycometabolic profile and health-related quality of life. Endocr Connect 2018;7(1):211–9.
19. Isidori AM, Venneri MA, Graziadio C, et al. Effect of once-daily, modified-release hydrocortisone versus standard glucocorticoid therapy on metabolism and innate immunity in patients with adrenal insufficiency (DREAM): a single-blind, randomised controlled trial. Lancet Diabetes Endocrinol 2018;6(3):173–85.
20. Nilsson AG, Bergthorsdottir R, Burman P, et al. Long-term safety of once-daily, dual-release hydrocortisone in patients with adrenal insufficiency: a phase 3b, open-label, extension study. Eur J Endocrinol 2017;176(6):715–25.
21. Lovas K, Loge JH, Husebye ES. Subjective health status in Norwegian patients with Addison's disease. Clin Endocrinol (Oxf) 2002;56(5):581–8.

22. Erichsen MM, Lovas K, Skinningsrud B, et al. Clinical, immunological, and genetic features of autoimmune primary adrenal insufficiency: observations from a Norwegian registry. J Clin Endocrinol Metab 2009;94(12):4882–90.
23. Didriksen NM, Saevik AB, Sortland LS, Oksnes M, Husebye ES. Sex-specific limitations in physical health in primary adrenal insufficiency. Front Endocrinol (Lausanne) 2021;12:718660.
24. Hahner S, Loeffler M, Fassnacht M, et al. Impaired subjective health status in 256 patients with adrenal insufficiency on standard therapy based on cross-sectional analysis. J Clin Endocrinol Metab 2007;92(10):3912–22.
25. Li D, Genere N, Behnken E, et al. Determinants of self-reported health outcomes in adrenal insufficiency: a multisite survey study. J Clin Endocrinol Metab 2021; 106(3):e1408–19.
26. Lindsay JR, Nansel T, Baid S, Gumowski J, Nieman LK. Long-term impaired quality of life in Cushing's syndrome despite initial improvement after surgical remission. J Clin Endocrinol Metab 2006;91(2):447–53.
27. van Aken MO, Pereira AM, Biermasz NR, et al. Quality of life in patients after long-term biochemical cure of Cushing's disease. J Clin Endocrinol Metab 2005;90(6): 3279–86.
28. Kauppinen-Makelin R, Sane T, Sintonen H, et al. Quality of life in treated patients with acromegaly. J Clin Endocrinol Metab 2006;91(10):3891–6.
29. Dekkers OM, Biermasz NR, Smit JW, et al. Quality of life in treated adult craniopharyngioma patients. Eur J Endocrinol 2006;154(3):483–9.
30. Andela CD, Scharloo M, Pereira AM, Kaptein AA, Biermasz NR. Quality of life (QoL) impairments in patients with a pituitary adenoma: a systematic review of QoL studies. Pituitary 2015;18(5):752–76.
31. Wagenmakers MA, Netea-Maier RT, Prins JB, Dekkers T, den Heijer M, Hermus AR. Impaired quality of life in patients in long-term remission of Cushing's syndrome of both adrenal and pituitary origin: a remaining effect of long-standing hypercortisolism? Eur J Endocrinol 2012;167(5):687–95.
32. Sagar R, Mackie S, Morgan AW, Stewart P, Abbas A. Evaluating tertiary adrenal insufficiency in rheumatology patients on long-term systemic glucocorticoid treatment. Clin Endocrinol (Oxf) 2021;94(3):361–70.
33. Borresen SW, Klose M, Baslund B, et al. Adrenal insufficiency is seen in more than one-third of patients during ongoing low-dose prednisolone treatment for rheumatoid arthritis. Eur J Endocrinol 2017;177(4):287–95.
34. Borresen SW, Thorgrimsen TB, Jensen B, et al. Adrenal insufficiency in prednisolone-treated patients with polymyalgia rheumatica or giant cell arteritis-prevalence and clinical approach. Rheumatology (Oxford) 2020;59(10):2764–73.
35. Joseph RM, Hunter AL, Ray DW, Dixon WG. Systemic glucocorticoid therapy and adrenal insufficiency in adults: A systematic review. Semin Arthritis Rheum 2016; 46(1):133–41.
36. Mehta P, Meeran K, Macphie E, et al. Variability in counselling for adrenal insufficiency in COVID-19 and beyond: a survey of rheumatology practice. Lancet Rheumatol 2021;3(2):e92–4.
37. Johannsson G, Bergthorsdottir R, Nilsson AG, Lennernas H, Hedner T, Skrtic S. Improving glucocorticoid replacement therapy using a novel modified-release hydrocortisone tablet: a pharmacokinetic study. Eur J Endocrinol 2009;161(1): 119–30.
38. Giordano R, Guaraldi F, Marinazzo E, et al. Improvement of anthropometric and metabolic parameters, and quality of life following treatment with dual-release hydrocortisone in patients with Addison's disease. Endocrine 2016;51(2):360–8.

39. Whitaker M, Debono M, Huatan H, Merke D, Arlt W, Ross RJ. An oral multiparticulate, modified-release, hydrocortisone replacement therapy that provides physiological cortisol exposure. Clin Endocrinol (Oxf) 2014;80(4):554–61.
40. Jones CM, Mallappa A, Reisch N, et al. Modified-release and conventional glucocorticoids and diurnal androgen excretion in congenital adrenal hyperplasia. J Clin Endocrinol Metab 2017;102(6):1797–806.
41. Mallappa A, Sinaii N, Kumar P, et al. A phase 2 study of Chronocort, a modified-release formulation of hydrocortisone, in the treatment of adults with classic congenital adrenal hyperplasia. J Clin Endocrinol Metab 2015;100(3):1137–45.
42. Gagliardi L, Nenke MA, Thynne TR, et al. Continuous subcutaneous hydrocortisone infusion therapy in Addison's disease: a randomized, placebo-controlled clinical trial. J Clin Endocrinol Metab 2014;99(11):4149–57.
43. Lovas K, Husebye ES. Continuous subcutaneous hydrocortisone infusion in Addison's disease. Eur J Endocrinol 2007;157(1):109–12.
44. Mallappa A, Nella AA, Sinaii N, et al. Long-term use of continuous subcutaneous hydrocortisone infusion therapy in patients with congenital adrenal hyperplasia. Clin Endocrinol (Oxf) 2018;89(4):399–407.
45. Oksnes M, Bjornsdottir S, Isaksson M, et al. Continuous subcutaneous hydrocortisone infusion versus oral hydrocortisone replacement for treatment of addison's disease: a randomized clinical trial. J Clin Endocrinol Metab 2014;99(5):1665–74.
46. Harbeck B, Kropp P, Monig H. Effects of short-term nocturnal cortisol replacement on cognitive function and quality of life in patients with primary or secondary adrenal insufficiency: a pilot study. Appl Psychophysiol Biofeedback 2009;34(2):113–9.
47. Werumeus Buning J, Brummelman P, Koerts J, et al. Hydrocortisone dose influences pain, depressive symptoms and perceived health in adrenal insufficiency: a randomized controlled trial. Neuroendocrinology 2016;103(6):771–8.
48. Werumeus Buning J, Brummelman P, Koerts J, et al. The effects of two different doses of hydrocortisone on cognition in patients with secondary adrenal insufficiency–results from a randomized controlled trial. Psychoneuroendocrinology 2015;55:36–47.
49. Gruber LM, Bancos I. Secondary adrenal insufficiency: recent updates and new directions for diagnosis and management. Endocr Pract 2022;28(1):110–7.
50. Arlt W. The approach to the adult with newly diagnosed adrenal insufficiency. J Clin Endocrinol Metab 2009;94(4):1059–67.
51. Arlt W, Callies F, Allolio B. DHEA replacement in women with adrenal insufficiency–pharmacokinetics, bioconversion and clinical effects on well-being, sexuality and cognition. Endocr Res 2000;26(4):505–11.
52. Hunt PJ, Gurnell EM, Huppert FA, et al. Improvement in mood and fatigue after dehydroepiandrosterone replacement in Addison's disease in a randomized, double blind trial. J Clin Endocrinol Metab 2000;85(12):4650–6.
53. Gurnell EM, Hunt PJ, Curran SE, et al. Long-term DHEA replacement in primary adrenal insufficiency: a randomized, controlled trial. J Clin Endocrinol Metab 2008;93(2):400–9.
54. Alkatib AA, Cosma M, Elamin MB, et al. A systematic review and meta-analysis of randomized placebo-controlled trials of DHEA treatment effects on quality of life in women with adrenal insufficiency. J Clin Endocrinol Metab 2009;94(10):3676–81.
55. Thompson RD, Carlson M, Thompson RD, Carlson M. Liquid chromatographic determination of dehydroepiandrosterone (DHEA) in dietary supplement products. J AOAC Int 2000;83(4):847–57.

56. Wierman ME, Kiseljak Vasilliades K. Should DHEA be administered to women? J Clin Endocrinol Metab 2022;7. https://doi.org/10.1210/clinem/dgac130.
57. Castinetti F, Sahnoun M, Albarel F, et al. An observational study on adrenal insufficiency in a French tertiary centre: real life versus theory. Ann Endocrinol *(Paris)* 2015;76(1):1–8.
58. Claessen K, Andela CD, Biermasz NR, Pereira AM. Clinical unmet needs in the treatment of adrenal crisis: importance of the patient's perspective. Front Endocrinol (Lausanne) 2021;12:701365.
59. Hahner S, Spinnler C, Fassnacht M, et al. High incidence of adrenal crisis in educated patients with chronic adrenal insufficiency: a prospective study. J Clin Endocrinol Metab 2015;100(2):407–16.
60. Allolio B. Extensive expertise in endocrinology. Adrenal crisis. Eur J Endocrinol 2015;172(3):R115–24.
61. Smans LC, Van der Valk ES, Hermus AR, Zelissen PM. Incidence of adrenal crisis in patients with adrenal insufficiency. Clin Endocrinol (Oxf) 2016;84(1):17–22.
62. White K, Arlt W. Adrenal crisis in treated Addison's disease: a predictable but under-managed event. Eur J Endocrinol 2010;162(1):115–20.
63. Erichsen MM, Lovas K, Fougner KJ, et al. Normal overall mortality rate in Addison's disease, but young patients are at risk of premature death. Eur J Endocrinol 2009;160(2):233–7.
64. Baud D, Qi X, Nielsen-Saines K, Musso D, Pomar L, Favre G. Real estimates of mortality following COVID-19 infection. Lancet Infect Dis 2020;20(7):773.
65. Bancos I, Hazeldine J, Chortis V, et al. Primary adrenal insufficiency is associated with impaired natural killer cell function: a potential link to increased mortality. Eur J Endocrinol 2017;176(4):471–80.
66. Isidori AM, Arnaldi G, Boscaro M, et al. COVID-19 infection and glucocorticoids: update from the Italian Society of Endocrinology Expert Opinion on steroid replacement in adrenal insufficiency. J Endocrinol Invest 2020;43(8):1141–7.
67. Arlt W, Baldeweg SE, Pearce SHS, Simpson HL. Endocrinology in the time of Covid-19: Management of adrenal insufficiency. Eur J Endocrinol 2020;183(1): G25–32.

Symptoms of Late-Onset Hypogonadism in Men

Peter J. Snyder, MD

KEYWORDS

• Testosterone • Hypogonadism • Late-onset hypogonadism

KEY POINTS

- Hypogonadism that occurs due to pituitary or testicular disease, sometimes called "classical hypogonadism," results in unequivocally low testosterone levels and in well-recognized symptoms that respond dramatically to the replacement of testosterone.
- Hypogonadism that occurs for no discernible reason other than aging, called late-onset hypogonadism, occurs in a small percentage of older men.
- The degree of hypogonadism and the corresponding symptoms are less pronounced in men with late-onset hypogonadism than in men who have classical hypogonadism, who typically have more severe hypogonadism.
- Testosterone treatment of men who have late-onset hypogonadism increases all aspects of self-reported sexual function and also improves, to a small degree, mood, depressive symptoms, and self-reported walking ability.
- Testosterone treatment of men who have late-onset hypogonadism does not improve vitality.

INTRODUCTION

The symptoms that result from male hypogonadism of a moderate to severe degree as a consequence of recognizable diseases of the pituitary or testes are well known and readily recognized. They include, especially, low libido, energy, and motivation, which improve dramatically when the patient's testosterone is raised to normal by treatment with testosterone.[1]

Men who have less severe hypogonadism, and for no discernible reason other than age, often called late-onset hypogonadism, may have similar symptoms but to a lesser degree. Because these symptoms can also be caused by many other medical and nonmedical conditions, it is essential to document that a patient's serum testosterone concentration is unequivocally and repeatedly low before ascribing the symptoms to hypogonadism.

Division of Endocrinology, Diabetes and Metabolism, Perelman School of Medicine, University of Pennsylvania, 12-135 Smilow Center for Translational Research, 3400 Civic Center Boulevard, Philadelphia, PA 19104, USA
E-mail address: pjs@pennmedicine.upenn.edu

Endocrinol Metab Clin N Am 51 (2022) 755–760
https://doi.org/10.1016/j.ecl.2022.04.001

SYMPTOMS OF HYPOGONADISM

Sexual Symptoms

A few recent studies have evaluated sexual symptoms in men with late-onset hypogonadism.

The European Male Aging Study–This prospective, observational study evaluated 3369 men ages 40 to 79 years at eight centers in Europe.[2] Serum concentrations of total and free testosterone were measured in the morning. Sexual symptoms were assessed by a questionnaire that was developed and validated for this study (European Male Aging Study–Sexual Function Questionnaire) that included 4 areas of sexual function: overall sexual functioning, masturbation, sexual functioning-distress, and change in sexual functioning.[3] Three sexual symptoms–decreased frequency of morning erections, decreased sexual desire, and erectile dysfunction–were found to have a syndromic association with low serum testosterone, although many men whose testosterone levels were normal also had sexual symptoms. If the diagnosis of late-onset hypogonadism were to require these 3 sexual symptoms, a serum testosterone concentration less than 11 nM (317 ng/dL) and a free testosterone less than 220 PM (63.4 pg/mL), the prevalence of hypogonadism in this population would be 0.1% in men 40 to 49 years and 5.1% in men 70 to 79 years. These data demonstrate that although symptoms suggesting hypogonadism in older men are common, actual hypogonadism is uncommon.

Trial of 2% Testosterone Gel–A clinical trial of its 2% testosterone gel in hypogonadal men, mostly due to late-onset hypogonadism or comorbidities, to determine the effect on sexual interest and energy.[4] The 715 men, whose baseline serum testosterone was 202 ng/dL, were randomized to receive testosterone or placebo gel for 12 weeks. In the subset of men who had low sexual drive at baseline, testosterone treatment of 311 men increased sexual interest significantly more than did placebo treatment of 308 men.

The Testosterone Trials–The Testosterone Trials (TTrials) were a group of 7 coordinated trials to determine if testosterone had any efficacy in older men with late-onset hypogonadism.[5] This condition was defined as a morning serum testosterone less than 275 ng/dL twice for no apparent reason other than age and suggestive symptoms. The TTrials enrolled 788 men whose mean baseline testosterone level was 232 ng/dL and allocated them to take testosterone or placebo gel for 1 year. One of the TTrials was the Sexual Function Trial, which enrolled 470 men who reported diminished sexual desire. Sexual activity was evaluated by the Psychosexual Daily Questionnaire, for which participants answered questions about all aspects of sexual activity by interactive voice response daily for 7 consecutive days every 3 months. Sexual interest was evaluated by the Derogatis Sexual Function Inventory and erectile function by the International Index of Erectile Function. Testosterone treatment significantly improved all aspects of sexual function, sexual activity (**Fig. 1**), and sexual interest more than erectile function. Testosterone improved all types of sexual activity, from flirting to intercourse (**Fig. 2**).[6] The magnitude of the increases in the serum levels of testosterone and estradiol were significantly associated with the magnitude of the improvements in sexual activity and interest but not erectile function.

Vitality/Fatigue

Trial of 2 percent testosterone gel–In the randomized trial of the 2% testosterone gel described above,[4] participants self-administered, via a hand-held device, 2 questions, each an 11-point Likert scale energy questionnaire, twice a day for a week. Of the subset of hypogonadal men (318 in each arm) who also had low energy, testosterone

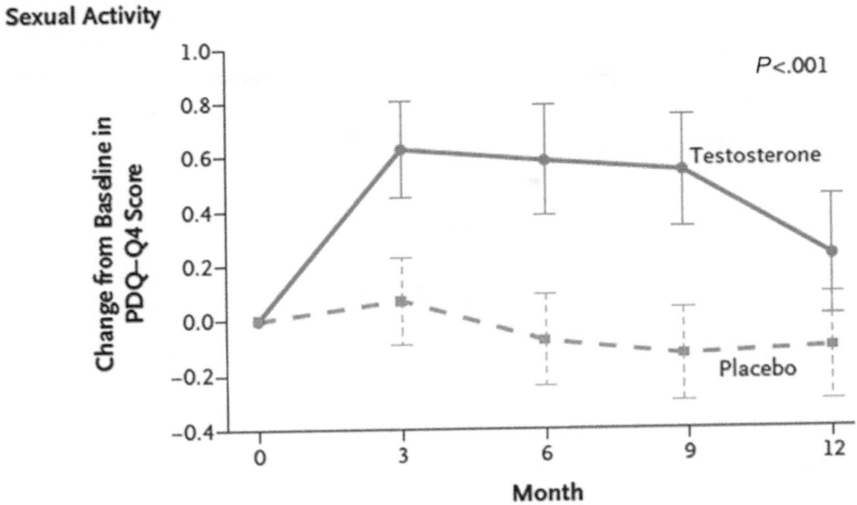

No. at Risk

	0	3	6	9	12
Testosterone	230	205	208	205	193
Placebo	229	198	189	190	193

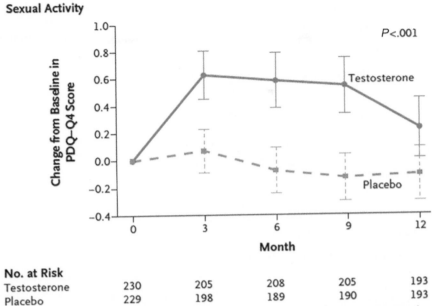

Fig. 1. The effect of testosterone compared with placebo treatment for 1 year on sexual activity, as measured by question 4 of the Psychosexual Daily Questionnaire (PDQ-Q4). (*From* Snyder PJ, Bhasin S, Cunningham GR, et al. Effects of Testosterone Treatment in Older Men. *N Engl J Med*. 2016;374(7):611-624.)

treatment increased energy more than did placebo, but the increase did not reach the prespecified significance level of $P < .01$.

The Testosterone Trials–In the Vitality Trial of The Testosterone Trials, the Facit-Fatigue Scale, a 40-item questionnaire. was used to evaluate energy at one end of the scale to fatigue at the other. Testosterone treatment of 236 men with low vitality did not increase their vitality significantly more than placebo treatment of 238 men with low vitality.[5] Testosterone treatment did increase vitality to a small degree (effect size 0.14) as assessed by the vitality component of the SF36 instrument. In addition, men treated with testosterone were significantly more likely to report, on a five-point scale, that their energy was better than were men treated with placebo.

Mood

Men who participated in the Vitality Trial of The Testosterone Trials were assessed for mood by the Positive and Negative Affect Scales,[5] a questionnaire that asks subjects to rate themselves from 1 to 5 with regard to 20 emotions. Testosterone treatment, compared with placebo, significantly increased positive affect to a small degree (effect size 0.14) and significantly decreased negative affect to a small degree (effect size.−0.18) (**Tables 1** and **2**). Testosterone treatment also decreased depressive symptoms to a small degree (effect size −0.18), as assessed by the PHQ depression score.

Self-Perception of Physical Function

In The Testosterone Trials, self-reported physical function was assessed by the physical function scale of the SF36 instrument (**Table 2**) and by a global impression of

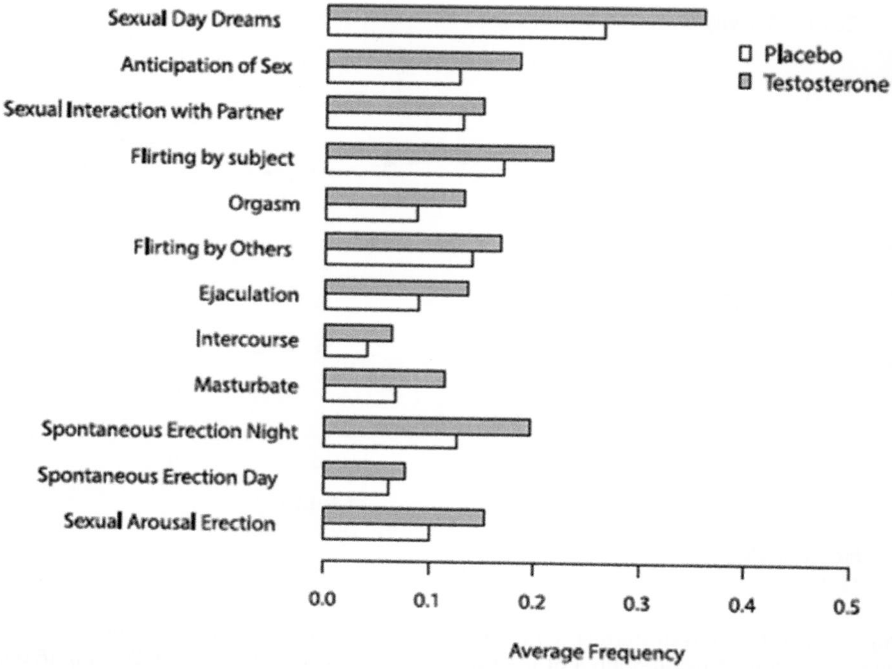

Fig. 2. Effect of testosterone compared with placebo treatment for 1 year on different aspects of sexual activity, as assessed by question 4 of the Psychosexual Daily Questionnaire. (*From* Cunningham GR, Stephens-Shields AJ, Rosen RC, et al. Testosterone Treatment and Sexual Function in Older Men With Low Testosterone Levels. J Clin Endocrinol Metab. 2016;101(8):3096-3104.)

change question about walking.[5] The physical function scale (PF10) of the SF36 is comprised of 10 questions about physical activity, ranging from light (bathing and dressing) to moderate (climbing stairs) to strenuous (running). Testosterone treatment was associated with a significantly increased PF10 score to a small degree (effect size 0.15). The global impression of change question the men were asked was, "Since the

Table 1
The effect of testosterone compared with placebo treatment for 1 year on mood, as assessed by the positive and negative affect scales of the PANAS instrument, and on depressive symptoms, as assessed by the patient health questionnaire-9 (PHQ-9)

Test	Treatment	Baseline	Change at 12 months	Treatment Effect	*P* Value
Positive Affect[1]	Testosterone	15.3 ± 3.2	0.7 ± 3.9	0.47 (0.02–0.92)	.04
	Placebo	15.4 ± 3.5	0.2 ± 3.2		
Negative Affect[2]	Testosterone	7.5 ± 2.7	−0.6 ± 2.1	−0.49 (−0.79–0.19)	<.001
	Placebo	7.4 ± 2.8	−0.1 ± 2.6		
PHQ-9[3]	Testosterone	6.6 ± 4.0	−1.8 ± 3.7	−0.72 (−0.30–0.06)	.004
	Placebo	6.6 ± 4.0	−1.1 ± 3.8		

Adapted from Snyder PJ, Bhasin S, Cunningham GR, et al. Effects of Testosterone Treatment in Older Men. *N Engl J Med*. 2016;374(7):611-624.

Table 2
The effect of testosterone compared with placebo treatment for 1 year on walking distance and the physical function component (PF-10) of the SF-36 questionnaire

Test	Treatment	Baseline	Change at Month 12	*P* Value
Walking Distance (m)	Testosterone	387.0 ± 81.7	6.69	.007
	Placebo	387.0 ± 83.7	1.50	
PF-10 Score	Testosterone	71.2 ± 20.2	4.3 ± 16.9	.002
	Placebo	69.7 ± 21.2	1.3 ± 16.9	

Adapted from Snyder PJ, Bhasin S, Cunningham GR, et al. Effects of Testosterone Treatment in Older Men. *N Engl J Med*. 2016;374(7):611-624.

beginning of the trial, is your walking much better, a little better, unchanged, a little worse, or much worse." Again, testosterone was associated with a significant improvement in the men's self-reported assessment of their walking ability.

DIAGNOSIS OF HYPOGONADISM IN MEN WHO HAVE SYMPTOMS

Although the studies above demonstrate that testosterone treatment for men who have late-onset hypogonadism improves the sexual, physical, and mood symptoms of this condition, most men who have these symptoms are not hypogonadal and therefore will not benefit from testosterone treatment. A striking, although not surprising, finding of the European Male Aging Study was that there were minimal differences between the mean serum testosterone levels in men who had symptoms suggestive of hypogonadism and men who did not have symptoms.[2] It is, therefore, of critical importance that the diagnosis of hypogonadism be clearly established before concluding that it is the cause of the symptoms. The diagnosis should be made by following the clinical guidelines of the Endocrine Society, which call for finding the serum testosterone concentration subnormal in the early morning on 3 occasions.[7] Measurement of total testosterone is usually sufficient, but because increased adiposity decreases sex hormone-binding globulin (SHBG) and therefore total testosterone, free testosterone should be measured by equilibrium dialysis in men who are overweight or obese. If the testosterone is unequivocally low, a specific cause should be sought.

TREATMENT OF HYPOGONADAL MEN

If a man is unequivocally hypogonadal due to an identifiable pituitary or testicular disease, testosterone should be replaced with the expectation that any symptoms of hypogonadism will probably improve. If, however, a man is hypogonadal for no apparent reason than age, that is, he has late-onset hypogonadism; there are 2 major issues with regard to treatment. One issue is that although testosterone treatment of men who have unequivocal late-onset hypogonadism has clear benefits, such as improvements in symptoms described above, and increases hemoglobin[8] and bone mineral density,[9] the risks of this treatment are not yet known, because no trial to date has been large enough or long enough to establish risk. The other issue is that the FDA specifically excludes late-onset hypogonadism from its approval of testosterone preparations.[10] The individual physician, therefore, must therefore decide for each whether or not to treat each hypogonadal man. Given the present state of knowledge and the current regulatory guidance, this author prescribes testosterone for men who have late-onset hypogonadism only if they have symptoms of hypogonadism and have a serum testosterone concentration that is reproducibly less than 200 ng/dL, a criterion that is more stringent than for men who are hypogonadal due to recognizable pituitary or testicular disease.

CLINICS CARE POINT

- Testosterone treatment of men with late-onset hypogonadism increases libido, sexual activity, hemoglobin, and bone mineral density, but the risks are unknown, so this author recommends treatment only if the symptoms are severe and the serum testosterone concentration is less than 200 ng/dL.

ACKNOWLEDGMENTS

The Testosterone Trials were supported by grants from the NIA (AG030644) and from AbbVie.

DISCLOSURE

The author has nothing to disclose.

REFERENCES

1. Snyder PJ, Peachey H, Berlin JA, et al. Effects of testosterone replacement in hypogonadal men. J Clin Endocrinol Metab 2000;85(8):2670–7. Available at: http://www.ncbi.nlm.nih.gov/htbin-post/Entrez/query?db=m&form=6&dopt=r&uid=10946864.
2. Wu FC, Tajar A, Beynon JM, et al. Identification of late-onset hypogonadism in middle-aged and elderly men. N Engl J Med 2010;363(2):123–35.
3. O'Connor DB, Corona G, Forti G, et al. Assessment of sexual health in aging men in Europe: development and validation of the European Male Ageing Study sexual function questionnaire. J Sex Med 2008;5(6):1374–85.
4. Brock G, Heiselman D, Maggi M, et al. Effect of testosterone solution 2% on testosterone concentration, sex drive and energy in hypogonadal men: results of a placebo controlled study. J Urol 2016;195(3):699–705.
5. Snyder PJ, Bhasin S, Cunningham GR, et al. Effects of testosterone treatment in older men. N Engl J Med 2016;374(7):611–24.
6. Cunningham GR, Stephens-Shields AJ, Rosen RC, et al. Testosterone treatment and sexual function in older men with low testosterone levels. J Clin Endocrinol Metab 2016;101(8):3096–104.
7. Bhasin S, Brito JP, Cunningham GR, et al. Testosterone therapy in men with hypogonadism: an endocrine society clinical practice guideline. J Clin Endocrinol Metab 2018;103(5):1715–44.
8. Snyder PJ, Kopperdahl DL, Stephens-Shields AJ, et al. Effect of testosterone treatment on volumetric bone density and strength in older men with low testosterone: a controlled clinical trial. JAMA Intern Med 2017;177(4):471–9.
9. Roy CN, Snyder PJ, Stephens-Shields AJ, et al. Association of testosterone levels with anemia in older men: a controlled clinical trial. JAMA Intern Med 2017;177(4):480–90.
10. Nguyen TV, Eisman JA, Kelly PJ, et al. Risk factors for osteoporotic fractures in elderly men. Am J Epidemiol 1996;144:255–63.

The Patient Experience of Thyroid Cancer

Susan C. Pitt, MD, MPHS[a], Kyle Zanocco, MD, MS[b], Cord Sturgeon, MD, MS[c,*]

KEYWORDS

• Thyroid cancer • Quality of life • Patient reported outcomes • Cancer diagnosis

KEY POINTS

- In 2019, the United States thyroid cancer survivor population was estimated to be more than 900,000.
- The quality of life (QOL) in the thyroid cancer survivor population is lower than the general population and lower than that of many other cancer survivor groups in some domains.
- Surgical and other treatment complications have a large negative impact of QOL.
- Mitigation efforts to improve QOL include renaming some low-risk cancers, reducing the extent of surgery, limiting the use of radioiodine, and active surveillance strategies.
- Prospective studies are needed to examine the short-term and long-term QOL impacts of these mitigation strategies.

INTRODUCTION

During the last decade, research on patient reported outcomes for thyroid cancer has increased almost exponentially. Early studies focused largely on survivorship and clinical outcomes of thyroidectomy and radioactive iodine (RAI) and demonstrated the need to improve our understanding of short-term and long-term quality of life (QOL) in this population. Several measures of QOL specific to patients with thyroid cancer have been developed to understand their unique, nuanced experience.[1,2] Many early study designs relied on retrospective, cross-sectional survey data.[1,3–5] More recently, researchers have expanded the inquiry to include prospective, qualitative studies using semistructured interviews or focus groups, discrete choice experiments (some with hypothetical designs), mixed-method evaluations, and more.[6–19] As a result, our understanding of how patients experience treatment effects, symptom burden, and other psychosocial issues following diagnosis and treatment of thyroid cancer

[a] Department of Surgery, University of Michigan Taubman 2920F, 1500 East Medical Center Drive, Ann Arbor, MI 48109, USA; [b] Department of Surgery, University of California Los Angeles, CHS 72-222, 10833 Le Conte Avenue, Los Angeles, CA 90095, USA; [c] Department of Surgery, Northwestern University, 676 North Saint Claire Street, Suite 650, Chicago, IL 60611, USA
* Corresponding author.
E-mail address: csturgeo@nm.org

Endocrinol Metab Clin N Am 51 (2022) 761–780
https://doi.org/10.1016/j.ecl.2022.04.002
endo.theclinics.com

Abbreviations	
WHOQOL-BREF	World Health Organization Quality of Life
PTH	Parathyroid hormone
RHRQOL	Health-related quality of life
EORTC QLQ	European Organization for the Research and Treatment of Cancer Quality of Life Questionnaire
CESQIP	Collaborative Endocrine Surgery Quality Improvement Program
PROFILES	Patient Reported Outcomes Following Initial treatment and Long term Evaluation of Survivorship
MFI-20	Multidimensional Fatigue Inventory
PTC	Papillary thyroid carcinoma

has expanded greatly. However, few have used randomized controlled designs and generated level one evidence to understand the effect of different treatments on patient experience and QOL.[20]

This review focuses on the patient experience with thyroid cancer and almost exclusively discusses the experience of those with differentiated thyroid cancer (papillary, follicular, and Hürthle cell). The experience of those with more aggressive thyroid cancers, such as medullary or anaplastic, likely differs because of the different extent of recommended initial treatment, worse prognosis, and different adjunct treatments such as chemotherapy or radiation. For those patients with differentiated thyroid cancer, particularly those that are low-risk, the treatment paradigm in recent years has expanded to a wider range from active surveillance to total thyroidectomy with or without central neck dissection, which requires a higher level of shared decision-making and understanding of the patients' goals and priorities with respect to treatment.[21–23] The review is organized chronologically to follow patients' thyroid cancer experience with initial diagnosis, management, and finally survivorship.

THE DIAGNOSIS PHASE

A patient's experience with thyroid cancer is frequently heralded by a seemingly innocuous discovery such as an asymptomatic thyroid nodule found on imaging performed for another reason, a palpable or visible mass detected on physical examination, or a lump casually noticed by the patient. Most thyroid nodules are nonmalignant. Regardless, for some patients the thought of an abnormal growth triggers a visceral response characterized by anxiety or worry over the possibility that the lump could be "the big C"—cancer.[13,24] Misbeliefs driving these negative emotions may derive from the fact that public knowledge about, and experience with, thyroid cancer is low, whereas the familiarity with the potential of dying from more common, more aggressive cancers such as lung, breast, or colorectal, is high. In addition, information available on the Internet about thyroid cancer may be perfunctory or out-of-date and may lack critical information patients need about the disease and treatment options.[25]

WHAT IS IN A NAME? THE SHIFT TO NONINVASIVE FOLLICULAR THYROID NEOPLASM WITH PAPILLARY-LIKE NUCLEAR FEATURES

Recent data show that 64% of the public automatically think of death when they hear the word "cancer." Despite the fact that most thyroid cancers are slow growing with excellent survival at 10 or 20 years, public perception is still quite negative with 35% thinking of death when they hear "thyroid cancer." A recent change in terminology for some low-risk follicular-patterned thyroid lesions was designed to address this. Research on erminology describing thyroid cancer has shown that terms such as "papillary lesion" or "abnormal cells" are less likely to cause anxiety compared with the descriptor "papillary hyroid cancer."[26] Interestingly, when alternative descriptors are used that eliminate the erm "cancer," people are also more likely to prefer nonsurgical management of their odule.[27] Renaming small, very low-risk thyroid cancers with terms that remove the "cancer" label was supported by a study involving community members in Australia.[28] This line of research provided excellent support for changing "encapsulated noninvasive ollicular variant of papillary thyroid cancer" to "noninvasive follicular thyroid neoplasm vith papillary-like nuclear features (NIFTP)," a decision that was made because of the ery low-risk and indolent nature of the lesion. Such changes have the potential to lecrease psychological and emotional distress in patients diagnosed with NIFTP, and lecrease the use of total thyroidectomy for small, indolent cancers.

IAGNOSIS IS ASSOCIATED WITH NEGATIVE EMOTIONS

Once a diagnosis of thyroid cancer is made, patients often experience increased egative emotions such as panic, shock, and fear similar to those diagnosed with ny other cancer, particularly more aggressive or deadly cancer.[12,29,30] Qualitative lata from semistructured interviews of patients diagnosed with low-risk thyroid can-er who have yet to undergo thyroidectomy demonstrate that these emotions are nderpinned by a sense of urgency to get the cancer out of their body as quickly as ossible.[12,29] Studies in patients newly diagnosed with cancer (as well as those under-oing treatment, survivors, and those with undiagnosed thyroid nodules) similarly lemonstrate that patients experience high levels of psychological or emotional listress in addition to sleep disturbance.[30–39] As a result, by the time the newly diag-osed patient is seen by a specialist, many are severely stressed. Some have misbe-efs that are difficult to dispel and may affect their perception of the appropriate extent f surgery or the implications of postoperative thyroid hormone replacement.

HE POWER OF PERSUASIVE TERMS

By the time patients newly diagnosed with thyroid cancer (or a thyroid cancer recur-ence) are seen in the office by a specialist, their experience may already be colored y negative emotions ranging from mild nervousness to full blown panic.[11,12,29,31,32] hese emotions have the potential to affect the patient–doctor interaction and ommunication and consequently affect decision-making.[40–42] Studies have shown at when discussing treatment alternatives with patients with low-risk thyroid cancer, hysicians commonly consider patients' level of anxiety. However, the physician may escribe outcomes of treatment in persuasive terms such as "worry" if the patient hooses active surveillance or "peace of mind" if the patient chooses total thyroidec-omy.[41,43] The use of anticipated emotional outcomes when deliberating between al-ernatives is known in the fields of behavioral economics and decision psychology to trongly influence behavior and choice.[44–46] Therefore, during this critical time in a pa-ent's cancer journey, it is imperative that physicians understand how their descrip-ons of the disease and potential outcomes, that may or may not ever be realized, fluence patient choice.

Studies have shown that in order to ease patients' negative emotions, many physi-ians use education and framing to reassure patients that their thyroid cancer diag-osis is unlikely to result in death.[42] Surprisingly, physicians are less likely to use irect expressions of empathy, such as stating, "I can see you are really stressed bout your new diagnosis of cancer. That is a very natural reaction. I hope I can pro-de you with some information that puts your mind at ease."[42] Physicians often emphasize that thyroid cancer is the "good cancer" and compare thyroid cancer to other more deadly cancers such as pancreas or adrenal cancer.[47–49] This "good cancer" term, although reassuring to some patients, has been shown to minimize the experience of other patients.[47] Therefore, in general, descriptors that emphasize positive long-term outcomes are more preferable.

THE MANAGEMENT PHASE

Drivers of Poor Quality of Life During the Management Phase

Historically, the 3 pillars of treatment of differentiated thyroid cancer have been surgery, radioiodine, and thyroid stimulating hormone (TSH)-suppressive doses of levothyroxine. Before active surveillance was popularized, approximately 96% of patients with differentiated thyroid cancer underwent surgery,[50] and about half of those received radioiodine as adjuvant therapy.[51] TSH-suppressive doses of levothyroxine were given to most patients after surgery. Accordingly, short-term and long-term complications from these 3 treatments should be examined in the most detail to identify treatment-related drivers of poor QOL.

The QOL of thyroid cancer patients can be significantly impacted by both the major and minor complications of these therapies. Patients who are diagnosed with differentiated thyroid cancer face several treatment options of varying degrees of aggressiveness (eg, hemithyroidectomy, total thyroidectomy with or without radioiodine ablation, active surveillance with deferred intervention) and varying risks of complication. An understanding of the potential impact of these treatments on QOL is essential for physicians who treat thyroid cancer, so they can help their patients make decisions about their initial management strategy. Numerous instruments have been used to measure those impacts.

Quality of Life Instruments for Thyroid Cancer Patients

Generic instruments

Generic instruments typically assess broad domains of physical, mental, and social function with questions that apply to the general population. Examples of generic QOL instruments used to study thyroid cancer patients include the SF-36 and patient-reported outcomes measurement information system (PROMIS)-29 questionnaires.[52,53] Scores from generic QOL instruments can be compared across disease states, allowing investigators to compare QOL of patients undergoing thyroid cancer treatment to patients being treated for other types of cancer.[54]

Disease-specific instruments

Disease-specific instruments are, as the name suggests, designed to measure how specific aspects of a disease affect QOL (eg, symptom severity or impact of treatment side effects on social life). Thyroid-specific patient reported outcome measure, health-related quality of life questionnaire for thyroid cancer survivors (THYCA-QoL), and the Voice Handicap Index (VHI) are all disease-specific instruments that have been used to study patients with thyroid cancer in the initial management phase.[55–57] Compared with the generic QOL instruments, disease-specific instruments allow for a more precise assessment of the symptoms encountered during thyroid cancer management. However, QOL scores from these instruments are not typically comparable to the general population.

Preference-based utility measures

Expressing patient QOL as a single utility score ranging from 0 (death) to 1 (perfect health) is useful for calculating quality adjusted life years in cost-effectiveness studies comparing the value of different medical interventions. Direct preference-based utility measures including rating scales, time-tradeoff scenarios, and the standard gamble method require individuals to choose between the health state under investigation and alternative health states.[58] In rating scale utility measurement, subjects typically are asked to rank their preferences on a visual analog scale. In time trade-off scenarios, individuals are asked to choose how much lifetime they would forego to be restored from the health state to perfect health. The standard gamble method asks individuals to choose between continuation of life in the current health state versus a gamble producing either a more or less favorable health state. All of these methods have been used to derive utility scores for the health states related to thyroid cancer management complications.[59–61]

Generic QOL instruments known as indirect preference-based utility measures incorporate econometric techniques to derive utility scores from generic QOL questionnaires.[62] Although considerably less labor intensive to administer, they produce less reliable utility estimates compared with the direct measurement techniques. Indirect measures including EuroQOL and EQ6d have been used to determine the QOL of patients with papillary thyroid cancer who underwent uncomplicated thyroidectomy.[63] Generic and disease-specific instruments that have been administered to thyroid cancer patients to study the impact of various treatments on QOL during the initial management phase are shown in **Table 1**.

Short-Term Quality of Life Changes After Uncomplicated Thyroid Cancer Surgery

All of the surgical therapies offered for thyroid cancer result in at least a short-term detriment to patients' QOL. Even the best-executed, uncomplicated procedure results in time away from work or normal routines. Successful operations also do not prevent patients from incurring substantial financial cost, postoperative pain, and alteration in appearance from the surgical scar. Shoulder and neck pain from patient positioning can also persist for several weeks. The standard anterior neck incision for thyroid cancer operations results in a scar that is initially prominent and then typically fades during a year or more of remodeling. Patients rate the cosmesis of thyroidectomy scars lower than their health-care providers using the same visual analog scale, suggesting that the personal experience of a neck scar has a negative impact on QOL.[64] Utility measurement of a new transverse cervical scar via the time tradeoff method showed a decrement of only 0.017, which is similar to many mild chronic disease states.[61]

Impact of Surgical Complications on Quality of Life

Recurrent laryngeal nerve injury

Injury to one of the recurrent laryngeal nerves (RLNs) can result in temporary or permanent unilateral vocal cord paralysis (UVCP) with diminished vocal quality and volume, an ineffective cough, and aspiration of thin liquids. The productivity of patients who depend on their voices at work is particularly affected by this complication. Generic and disease-specific assessments of patients with UVCP demonstrate general and voice-related impairment in QOL, specifically in the domains of physical and social functioning with a utility detriment estimated to be 11% to 37%.[60,61,65,66] Treatments for UVCP include vocal fold medialization procedures with office-based vocal fold injection of bulking agents or surgical placement of a permanent laryngeal implant. These interventions have been shown to improve QOL in affected patients with Voice-Related Quality of Life Measure scores increasing from preintervention "poor" or "fair" voice quality ratings to mostly "good" or "very good" following medialization.[65,67]

Table 1
Quality of life instruments used to assess patients with thyroid cancer undergoing initial management

Instrument	Number of Items	Conditions Studied
Generic QOL instruments		
Rand Medical Outcome Study Short Form Health Surveys (SF-12, SF-20, SF-36)[52]	12–36	RLN injury Hypoparathyroidism Hypothyroidism Active surveillance with deferred intervention for low-risk thyroid cancer
Abbreviated World Health Organization Quality of Life Scale-BREF[119]	26	Tracheostomy
Indirect preference based utility measures[a]	Various	Postoperative QOL without complications after treatment of papillary thyroid cancer
Disease specific QOL instruments		
Voice Handicap Index[57]	30	Recurrent nerve injury Dysphonia
Voice outcome survey[120]	5	Recurrent nerve injury Dysphonia
Voice-Related Quality of Life[65]	10	Recurrent nerve injury Dysphonia
Reflux symptoms index[121]	9	Dysphagia and dysphonia
Dermatology life Quality Index[122]	10	Thyroidectomy scar
Thyroid-specific patient reported outcome measure[123]	84	Postoperative hypothyroidism
Health-related quality of life questionnaire for thyroid cancer survivors[56]	24	Active surveillance with deferred intervention for low risk thyroid cancer
Fear of Progression Questionnaire[124]	43	Active surveillance with deferred intervention for low risk thyroid cancer
Xerostomia Quality of Life Scale[125]	15	Sialadenitis following radioiodine therapy
MD Anderson Dysphagia Inventory[126]	20	Sialadenitis following radioiodine therapy
University of Washington Quality of Life Instrument[127]	9	Sialadenitis following radioiodine therapy
Direct preference-based utility measures[b]	Various	Postthyroidectomy scar, hypoparathyroidism, hypothyroidism and RLN injury

[a] Include Short Form-12v2 (SF6D), EuroQol-5D (EQ5D), Health Utilities Index Mark 2 and 3 (HUI2, HUI3).[128–131]
[b] Include disease specific assessment of health states via rating scale, standard gamble, and time tradeoff techniques.[59–61]

Bilateral vocal cord paralysis (BVCP) due to injury to both RLNs during thyroidectomy is an exceedingly rare outcome that results in severe QOL changes with utility detriment estimates greater than 50%.[60,61] BVCP typically necessitates tracheostomy placement to allow airway patency. On the Abbreviated World Health Organization Quality of Life Scale-BREF, patients with a newly placed tracheostomy reported the most significant area of QOL detriment in the environmental domain, which includes perceptions of environmental safety, access to health services, and opportunities for leisure.[68] Surgical enlargement of the airway space with arytenoidectomy and posterior cordectomy can allow patients with BVCP to breathe normally without a tracheostomy. However, these procedures are at the expense of voice quality and have been shown to produce moderate dysphonia when posttreatment patients are evaluated with the VHI.[69,70]

Voice and swallowing impairment without recurrent nerve injury

Although recurrent nerve injury is relatively rare, most patients undergoing thyroid cancer surgery experience some degree of dysphonia and dysphagia during the first postoperative month, likely resulting from postoperative inflammation in the dissected thyroid bed and/or injury to the external branch of the superior laryngeal nerve (EBSLN). EBSLN injury results in vocal weakness, shortened phonation time, reduced vocal range, and detriment to singing voice, which decreases QOL measured by the VHI.[71,72] A study of swallowing impairment symptoms following surgery for papillary thyroid cancer in the absence of RLN injury demonstrated an 80% rate of patients reporting a globus sensation and subjective difficulty in swallowing; however, less than 10% of patients had videofluoroscopic findings suggestive of clinically significant dysphagia.[73] These symptoms persisted after 6 months in 17% of patients, suggesting that patients should be counseled about the possibility of subjective dysphagia following otherwise uncomplicated thyroid cancer surgery.

Hypoparathyroidism

Hypocalcemia resulting from devascularization and/or inadvertent excision of parathyroid tissue during total thyroidectomy is common in the immediate postoperative period, readily treatable with medication, and usually self-limited. Chronic hypoparathyroidism requiring lifelong calcium and vitamin D supplementation to maintain normocalcemia occurs in less than 2% of operations; however, this complication has been shown in several studies to negatively affect QOL in a degree that is similar to diabetes or chronic heart disease.[74] SF-36 scores in these patients are particularly worse than the general population in the vitality, physical functioning, and bodily pain domains.[75] Utility is decreased by chronic hypoparathyroidism by an estimated 10%; however, the underlying mechanism for this decrement is unclear.[61] Many thought that parathyroid hormone directly affects neurocognitive function because PTH acts on receptors in the brain and treatment with recombinant parathyroid hormone in eucalcemic hypoparathyroid patients has been found to significantly improve QOL.[76]

Early Postoperative Management

Radioiodine remnant ablation

In patients undergoing postoperative radioiodine therapy, QOL can be affected by both preablation thyroid hormone withdrawal and ablation-related side effects. The long half-life of levothyroxine requires discontinuation for up to 4 to 6 weeks to act on the hypothalamus-pituitary axis and increase endogenous TSH to facilitate uptake of RAI into remnant thyroid cells. Large negative effects in the physical and social functioning, role limitations, and energy domains of the SF-36 are observed before ablation among patients undergoing thyroid hormone withdrawal.[77] Utility decreases an estimated 20% during the withdrawal period.[78] Shortening the withdrawal period with liothyronine bridge therapy or eliminating it with administration of recombinant human TSH (rhTSH) can improve preablation QOL. Randomized controlled trials comparing preablation withdrawal versus rhTSH have shown consistently favorable differences in the social functioning and mental health SF-36 domains for patients who avoided withdrawal with rhTSH.[77,79]

RAI therapy often causes temporary side effects of neck pain, nausea, and swollen salivary glands. Approximately 20% of patients receiving RAI for thyroid cancer reported symptoms of salivary gland toxicity, including chronic sialadenitis or xerostomia, at 1 year following therapy.[80] High-dose RAI (>150 mCi) has been associated with reduction of the daily swallowing function domain of the MD Anderson Dysphagia Inventory and diminished QOL in the social, psychological, and pain domains of the University of Washington Quality of Life Instrument.[81]

Initial thyroid stimulating hormone suppression

Suppression of TSH with supraphysiologic doses of levothyroxine is generally recommended to decrease the risk of recurrent differentiated thyroid cancer, especially in patients at a high risk of recurrence with tumors exhibiting gross extrathyroidal extension or distant metastatic disease.[82] Initiation of suppressive therapy can cause subclinical or even overt thyrotoxicosis with side effects including menopause, osteoporosis, atrial fibrillation, and exacerbation of angina in patients with ischemic heart disease. Isolating the negative impact of subclinical thyrotoxicosis on QOL during the first months of TSH suppression is confounded by many other treatment-related factors; however, a subgroup analysis of patients with thyroid cancer on TSH suppression within the first year of treatment showed impairment of the mental, physical, emotional, social functioning, and vitality domains of the SF-36, suggesting that TSH suppression is at least transiently associated with diminished QOL.[83] In comparison, Hoftijzer and colleagues found no correlation between QOL and TSH level in their follow-up study of apparently cured patients.[3]

The Cancer Survivorship Phase

The survivorship phase overlaps all the other phases. It begins at the time of cancer diagnosis and continues through cancer treatment and until the end of life. Many patients with thyroid cancer are considered cancer-free at some point in their survivorship, and some will continue to live with cancer for the remainder of life but all will have been “cancer survivors.” The unique needs and concerns of cancer survivors are driven, in part, by the financial, physical, mental, and social burdens placed on them by the cancer and the treatments received.

Excluding carcinomas in situ and basal cell and squamous cell skin cancers, it was estimated that, in 2019, there were nearly 17 million cancer survivors living in the United States (US).[84] This is more than 5% of the roughly 330 million population of the US. The large size and longevity of this population should be heralded as a medical success, with the caveat that the overdiagnosis of clinically irrelevant subclinical cancers artificially inflates these statistics. Other causes for growth in the population of cancer survivors include earlier detection, better treatments, better supportive care, and an increase in cancer detection.

The fidelity of imaging studies is continuously improving, as is the sensitivity of modalities used for screening and surveillance of cancer. This contributes to the detection of more subclinical or early-stage cancers, as well as the overdiagnosis of some indolent carcinomas, such as papillary thyroid microcarcinoma. Better detection and better treatments partially explain the size of the cancer survivor population. Improvements in treatment and supportive care also lead to longer survival. Despite efforts to reduce overdiagnosis, all predictions agree that the cancer survivor population is expected to grow in concert with the growing and aging US population.

Despite a large population of cancer survivors in the US, there are major gaps in our understanding of survivorship.[85] Most of the survivorship research that has been done has been in breast cancer. For other cancers, there are significant gaps in understanding. Few cancers have been studied beyond 5 years, many studies lack good control populations, and there is a dearth of interventional studies.

The United States Thyroid Cancer Survivor Population

In 2019, it was estimated that there were more than 900,000 thyroid cancer survivors living in the US.[84,86] Approximately 78% were women.[84] The median age at diagnosis was 51 years.[86] In 2021, thyroid cancer represented 2.3% of all new cancer cases, we added an estimated 44,280 new cases and lost an estimated 2200 persons from the disease. Most cases of thyroid cancer are well-differentiated papillary or follicular in histology, which have a very good prognosis. Fewer than 5% of thyroid cancers are medullary or anaplastic types, with a poor prognosis. The long-term survival of patients with differentiated thyroid cancer is generally reported to be greater than 90% but based on the above numbers, less than one-half of 1% of the thyroid cancer survivor population dies annually of thyroid cancer. Given the large and growing size of this population of survivors and the expected duration of survival, extending the length of life for patients with differentiated thyroid cancer is not the primary concern; rather, it is necessary to focus on measures that improve health-related QOL.

Quality of Life in Thyroid Cancer Survivors

Several publications have documented the QOL reported by survivors of thyroid cancer and have examined predictors of poor QOL.[54,87–94] It seems intuitive that for patients with a highly curable cancer, the QOL indices should be close to normal, especially when many years have passed since diagnosis and treatment, and the patient is apparently cured. However, despite the favorable prognosis of thyroid cancer compared with other cancers, most researchers have found that thyroid cancer survivors have worse QOL than the general population and similar or worse QOL than survivors of other cancers. These findings have been similar across multiple populations regardless of decade or national health-care system.

Goswami and colleagues[54] found that thyroid cancer survivors had statistically significantly worse QOL than the general US population and worse anxiety, depression, fatigue, and sleep disturbance than other cancer survivors but less pain and greater physical function. Applewhite and colleagues[90] found that HRQOL in US thyroid cancer survivors was similar to that of patients with colon, glioma, breast, and gynecologic cancers. Goldfarb and Casillas[1] surveyed US adult thyroid cancer survivors and found that female survivors had worse SF-6D scores than the general population. Young adult (aged 17–39 years) survivors had a significantly different THYCA-QoL profile than older adult (aged >39 years) survivors or the general population. Younger survivors had more psychological issues but fewer neuromuscular or voice issues. They found that complaints related to neuromuscular symptoms, concentration, or anxiety along with the presence of a comorbidity predicted lower overall HRQOL in young adult survivors. A survey conducted in the United Kingdom found that thyroid cancer survivors had a lower QOL than the general population in the United Kingdom and lower than that of patients with breast, colon, or prostate cancer.[87] Furthermore, approximately half of those surveyed complained of financial stress, weight gain, and forgetfulness and approximately 75% complained of fatigue. Husson and colleagues[88] surveyed thyroid cancer survivors from a Dutch registry who were at least 2 years from diagnosis. They used EORTC-QLQ-C30 and

THYCA-QoL and found that thyroid cancer survivors had significantly lower QOL than the normative Dutch population. Specifically, they reported more chills, hot flashes, leg cramps, fatigue, and pain in the joints and muscles. Lee and colleagues[91] have similarly found that thyroid cancer survivors in Korea have lower QOL compared with the general Korean population and that anxiety, depression, and fatigue were the major contributors.

Drivers of Long-Term Poor Quality of Life in Thyroid Cancer Survivors

Surgical complications

As discussed above, surgical complications are associated with lower QOL, and permanent complications should be expected to have a more profound and lasting impact on QOL than temporary complications. Permanent RLN injury and permanent hypoparathyroidism are more common than once thought, particularly for lower volume surgeons, and in patients undergoing thyroidectomy for malignancy. In a report from the CESQIP database, among 623 patients undergoing thyroidectomy for papillary thyroid cancer by high-volume thyroid surgeons, there was a permanent vocal cord dysfunction rate of 1% and a permanent hypocalcemia rate of 2.1%.[95] Similarly, in a recent meta-analysis that evaluated thyroidectomy specifically for cancer, Wong and colleagues found the overall RLN injury rate of 3.5% and permanent RLN injury rate of 1.2%.[96] Rates of 1% to 2% for permanent complications are commonly quoted but may not reflect outcomes for the broader population of patients with thyroid cancer. Columbo and colleagues[97] in their single-institution series reported that total thyroidectomy was associated with a permanent hypoparathyroidism rate of 10% and an RLN injury rate of 7.2%. In a recent multi-institutional cohort of 1453 Spanish patients treated with total thyroidectomy for cancer, Diez and colleagues reported a postoperative hypoparathyroidism rate of 47% with a permanent hypoparathyroidism rate of 13%.[98] Surveys of thyroid cancer support groups also reveal higher rates of reported hypoparathyroidism and permanent voice change. The Thyroid Cancer Alliance survey of 2380 thyroid cancer survivors reported chronic postsurgical hypoparathyroidism and voice changes in 14% and 13%, respectively.[99]

Surgical complications in particular have a significant negative impact on QOL.[92,100] We recognize that some studies have shown no impact of RLN injury or hypoparathyroidism on QOL but these studies were likely underpowered to show a difference, especially if the rates of reported surgical complications are low and the population is relatively small.[3,94] Conversely, in cohorts of patients with higher rates of hypoparathyroidism or RLN injury, it is clear that these surgical complications are associated with significant impairment in QOL.[101] In an observational study of French patients with hypoparathyroidism, Frey and colleagues[102] reported statistically significantly reduced mental score ratios on the SF-36 as well as lower voice quality compared with controls in survivors with a median time since surgery of 6 years. In a multinational QOL study of thyroid cancer survivors using the EORTC-QLQ-C30, scores were significantly worse in 9 of 15 scales in those with hypoparathyroidism compared with those without. Further, hypoparathyroidism was found to be an independent predictor of worse QOL. Surveys of the Thyroid Cancer Survivors' Association have also revealed that symptoms of hypocalcemia, dysphonia, or dysphagia are statistically significantly associated with worse QOL.[92,100]

Mitigation of surgical risk

One strategy to mitigate the risks of RLN injury and hypoparathyroidism is to perform a thyroid lobectomy instead of a total thyroidectomy whenever feasible. Thyroid lobectomy obviates the risks of complete voice loss and tracheostomy from bilateral

RLN injury as well as the risk of hypoparathyroidism. Patient selection is critical because although there may be a higher rate of structural or biochemical response in some patients treated with total thyroidectomy, this improved response comes with a greater chance of surgical complications.[97] For patients with low-risk thyroid cancer, hemithyroidectomy decreases the chances of surgical morbidity and post-operative hypothyroidism while providing excellent long-term oncologic outcomes. QOL has been compared between patients who underwent hemithyroidectomy and total thyroidectomy for small, differentiated thyroid cancers in the first few months after surgery via content analysis of patient interview transcripts from the Queensland Australia Thyroid Cancer Study.[103] Study patients who had a total thyroidectomy were 1.5 times more likely to report a health-related QOL issue than those treated with hemithyroidectomy. Common QOL concerns that were more frequent in the total thyroidectomy group included fatigue and inconvenience of life-long medication therapy. Conversely, a small study from the PROFILES registry compared patients who underwent lobectomy or total thyroidectomy for cancer and found no statistically significant differences in any of the 15 EORTC-QLQ scales.[104] Also, Bongers and colleagues[105] surveyed 270 survivors of low-risk differentiated thyroid cancer and found no difference between QOL between those treated with total thyroidectomy or lobectomy. There was a higher rate of worry about recurrence in the lobectomy group.

Complications from radioiodine and thyroid stimulating hormone suppression

Complications from radioiodine and TSH suppression have received less attention than surgical complications and have been harder to recognize due to the longer temporal relationship between exposure and development of symptoms.[106] As discussed above, several studies have shown a correlation between thyroid hormone withdrawal for radioiodine scans or ablation and either distress or poor QOL.[89,107] Although some studies have shown no correlation between I-131 dose and QOL, most studies have not been designed with that endpoint in mind.[3] Studies of larger thyroid cancer survivor cohorts have demonstrated a relationship between QOL and specific complications of radioiodine such as xerostomia, dental caries, and sialadenitis.[92,100]

HOW DOES TIME SINCE TREATMENT IMPACT QUALITY OF LIFE?

Several studies have found that short-term QOL in thyroid cancer survivors is impaired but over time QOL improves.[3,83,100] Chen and colleagues[108] found significant differences in QOL at 1 and 3 months after surgery between patients with low-to-intermediate risk thyroid cancer who underwent either lobectomy or total thyroidectomy. However, these differences were no longer apparent at 6 or 12 months. Crevenna and colleagues[83] surveyed 150 thyroid cancer survivors with SF-36 and found that time since treatment was correlated with improved scores in multiple domains. Hoftijzer and colleagues[3] found that longer duration of cure was correlated with better scores on SF-36 and MFI-20. They calculated that duration of cure might need to be 20 years for thyroid cancer survivors to return to normal QOL compared with population-based controls. Pelttari and colleagues surveyed 341 thyroid cancer survivors from a single institution in Helsinki. Each was either stage 1 or 2 and on average were greater than 12 years from treatment. They found that in this cohort of long-term survivors, QOL was not different than that of the general Finnish population.[94] More work needs to be done to understand the relationship between QOL and time since treatment. The drivers of this relationship are not well understood but it is well recognized that over time many patients can reasonably accommodate to permanent surgical complications such as RLN injury. The elimination of surgical scar has received much attention in the past decade but rarely outside of the context of industry-supported projects. Administration of the Dermatology Life Quality Index to patients with thyroid cancer at a median interval of 1 year after thyroidectomy produced a mean score of 9, which is comparable to patients with psoriasis and severe atopic dermatitis.[109] Kurumety and colleagues surveyed 1710 thyroid cancer survivors and reported that the impact of scar on HRQOL seems to be mild and transient, and patients reported that the neck appearance returned to baseline at 2 years after surgery.[93]

FINANCIAL BURDEN

Perhaps one of the most surprising findings in the study of thyroid cancer survivors has been the observation that they have a disproportionate level of financial burden and higher rate of bankruptcy compared with other cancer survivors.[110,111] The explanation for this may lie in the fact that thyroid cancer affects a younger age group than most cancers,[112] and that this group often does not quality for Medicare. Health insurance affordability, ongoing expenses for treatment, lost wages, transportation costs, and employment consequences all contribute to financial toxicity. Importantly, financial distress and negative financial events have been shown to be associated with poor QOL in patients with thyroid cancer.[111]

WILL DEFERRED INTERVENTION OR ALTERNATIVE STRATEGIES IMPROVE QUALITY OF LIFE?

In the last 10 years, deferred intervention and active surveillance strategies have gained favor for select patients. These patients may avoid the risks of surgery and radioiodine but still have the burden of stress, doctors' visits, and surveillance. A recent survey of physicians treating thyroid cancer in the US in 2017 revealed that approximately 94% agree that active surveillance is appropriate for some patients but interestingly the majority (76%) would choose surgery for themselves for a <1 cm PTC.[113]

This is an area that is ripe for investigation. In one study, patients who underwent active surveillance for papillary microcarcinoma showed less neuromuscular, throat, and scar problems on THYCA-QoL compared with those who underwent hemithyroidectomy.[114] These benefits were realized without significantly worse Fear of Progression scores in the active surveillance group. Others have found more pervasive concerns about recurrence. Hedman and colleagues[115] surveyed 353 patients from the Swedish Cancer Registry who were 14 to 17 years from diagnosis and found that 48% were concerned about recurrence, and that this group had a worse HRQOL than those who were not concerned about recurrence.

Active surveillance has the potential to completely mitigate the surgical risks as long as the patient does not experience disease progression and subsequently require treatment of a more invasive tumor or more extensive disease. Fortunately, longitudinal studies have shown that for small low-risk papillary carcinomas, progression or development of clinically overt nodal metastases is uncommon.[116–118]

Percutaneous ablation techniques are now available but have been mostly used for benign disease. Only long-term studies will demonstrate the relative value of active surveillance or percutaneous techniques versus surgical treatment at the time of diagnosis. It is important to recognize that worry over recurrence has been shown to impact QOL and should be factored into treatment decisions.[105,115]

SUMMARY

The experience of patients with thyroid cancer evolves from the time they are initially diagnosed through management and survivorship. The experience of most patients with thyroid cancer is unique because they carry the "cancer" label, yet have an overall excellent prognosis. Treatment is also different than those with many other cancers because it does not typically include traditional cancer therapeutics such as chemotherapy and external beam radiation. Although measurement of patient reported outcomes has increased and improved dramatically during recent decades, scope for improvement in the experience of patients with thyroid cancer still exists.

CLINICS CARE POINTS

- Patients with newly diagnosed cancer are often severely stressed and may benefit from direct expressions of empathy. Remember to describe the treatments and potential outcomes in nonbiased yet compassionate terms.
- During the treatment phase, carefully consider the extent of surgical and medical treatments in order to mitigate potential reduction in quality of life from side effects or complications of the treatments received.
- Thyroid cancer survivors may have chronic complications from surgery, radioiodine, and thyroid stimulating hormone suppression. They are also particularly vulnerable to financial toxicity. These conditions should be screened for and addressed during longitudinal care.

DISCLOSURE

Dr S.C. Pitt receives funding from the NCI award #K08CA230204.

REFERENCES

1. Goldfarb M, Casillas J. Thyroid Cancer-Specific Quality of Life and Health-Related Quality of Life in Young Adult Thyroid Cancer Survivors. Thyroid 2016;26:923–32.
2. Roth EM, Lubitz CC, Swan JS, et al. Patient-Reported Quality-of-Life Outcome Measures in the Thyroid Cancer Population. Thyroid 2020;30:1414–31.
3. Hoftijzer HC, Heemstra KA, Corssmit EP, et al. Quality of life in cured patients with differentiated thyroid carcinoma. J Clin Endocrinol Metab 2008;93:200–3.
4. Goldfarb M, Casillas J. Unmet information and support needs in newly diagnosed thyroid cancer: comparison of adolescents/young adults (AYA) and older patients. J Cancer Surviv 2014;8:394–401.
5. Morley SGM. Support Needs and Survivorship Concerns of Thyroid Cancer Patients. Thyroid 2015;25:649–56.
6. Nickel B, Howard K, Brito JP, et al. Association of Preferences for Papillary Thyroid Cancer Treatment With Disease Terminology: A Discrete Choice Experiment. JAMA Otolaryngol Head Neck Surg 2018;144:887–96.
7. Ahmadi S, Gonzalez JM, Talbott M, et al. Patient Preferences Around Extent of Surgery in Low-Risk Thyroid Cancer: A Discrete Choice Experiment. Thyroid 2020;30:1044–52.
8. Sukpanich R, Sanglestsawai S, Seib CD, et al. The Influence of Cosmetic Concerns on Patient Preferences for Approaches to Thyroid Lobectomy: A Discrete Choice Experiment. Thyroid 2020;30:1306–13.

9. Davies L, Hendrickson CD, Hanson GS. Experience of US Patients Who Self-identify as Having an Overdiagnosed Thyroid Cancer: A Qualitative Analysis. JAMA Otolaryngol Head Neck Surg 2017;143(7):663–9.
10. Nickel B, Brito JP, Barratt A, et al. Clinicians' Views on Management and Terminology for Papillary Thyroid Microcarcinoma: A Qualitative Study. Thyroid 2017; 27:661–71.
11. Hedman C, Strang P, Djarv T, et al. Anxiety and Fear of Recurrence Despite a Good Prognosis: An Interview Study with Differentiated Thyroid Cancer Patients. Thyroid 2017;27(11):1417–23.
12. Nickel B, Brito JP, Moynihan R, et al. Patients' experiences of diagnosis and management of papillary thyroid microcarcinoma: a qualitative study. BMC Cancer 2018;18:242.
13. Pitt SC, Wendt E, Saucke MC, et al. A Qualitative Analysis of the Preoperative Needs of Patients With Papillary Thyroid Cancer. J Surg Res 2019;244:324–31.
14. Nickel B, Semsarian C, Moynihan R, et al. Public perceptions of changing the terminology for low-risk thyroid cancer: a qualitative focus group study. BMJ Open 2019;9:e025820.
15. Sawka AM, Goldstein DP, Brierley JD, et al. The impact of thyroid cancer and post-surgical radioactive iodine treatment on the lives of thyroid cancer survivors: a qualitative study. PLoS One 2009;4:e4191.
16. D'Agostino TA. A Qualitative Analysis of Medical Decision-Making and Illness Experience in Early-Stage Thyroid Cancer: The New School; 2015.
17. Park SH, Lee B, Lee S, et al. A qualitative study of women's views on overdiagnosis and screening for thyroid cancer in Korea. BMC Cancer 2015;15:858.
18. Fordham BA, Kerr C, de Freitas HM, et al. Health state utility valuation in radioactive iodine-refractory differentiated thyroid cancer. Patient Prefer Adherence 2015;9:1561–72.
19. Misra S, Meiyappan S, Heus L, et al. Patients' experiences following local-regional recurrence of thyroid cancer: a qualitative study. J Surg Oncol 2013; 108:47–51.
20. Pitt SC. Quality of Life, Patient-Reported Outcomes, and Extent of Surgery for Patients With Low- and Intermediate-Risk-Differentiated Thyroid Cancer. JAMA Surg 2022;157(3):209–10.
21. Pitt SC, Lubitz CC. Complex decision making in thyroid cancer: Costs and consequences–is less more? Surgery 2017;161:134–6.
22. McDow AD, Pitt SC. Extent of Surgery for Low-Risk Differentiated Thyroid Cancer. Surg Clin North Am 2019;99:599–610.
23. Pitt SC, Saucke MC. Novel Decision Support Interventions for Low-risk Thyroid Cancer. JAMA Otolaryngol Head Neck Surg 2020;146(11):1079–81.
24. Jensen CB, Saucke MC, Francis DO, et al. From Overdiagnosis to Overtreatment of Low-Risk Thyroid Cancer: A Thematic Analysis of Attitudes and Beliefs of Endocrinologists, Surgeons, and Patients. Thyroid 2020;30:696–703.
25. Doubleday AR, Novin S, Long KL, et al. Online Information for Treatment for Low-Risk Thyroid Cancer: Assessment of Timeliness, Content, Quality, and Readability. J Cancer Educ 2020;36(4):850–7.
26. Nickel B, Barratt A, McGeechan K, et al. Effect of a Change in Papillary Thyroid Cancer Terminology on Anxiety Levels and Treatment Preferences: A Randomized Crossover Trial. JAMA Otolaryngol Head Neck Surg 2018;144:867–74.
27. Chen H, Roberts JR, Ball DW, et al. Effective long-term palliation of symptomatic, incurable metastatic medullary thyroid cancer by operative resection. Ann Surg 1998;227:887–95.

28. Shih P, Nickel B, Degeling C, et al. Terminology Change for Small Low-Risk Papillary Thyroid Cancer As a Response to Overtreatment: Results from Three Australian Community Juries. Thyroid 2021;31(7):1067–75.
29. Pitt SC, Saucke MC, Wendt EM, et al. Patients' Reaction to Diagnosis with Thyroid Cancer or an Indeterminate Thyroid Nodule. Thyroid 2020;31(4):580–8.
30. Buchmann L, Ashby S, Cannon RB, et al. Psychosocial distress in patients with thyroid cancer. Otolaryngol Head Neck Surg 2015;152:644–9.
31. Pitt SC, Haymart MR. Breaking Down or Waking Up? Psychological Distress and Sleep Disturbance in Patients With Thyroid Nodules and Cancer. J Clin Endocrinol Metab 2021;106:e4278–80.
32. Jensen CB, Pitt SC. Patient perception of receiving a thyroid cancer diagnosis. Curr Opin Endocrinol Diabetes Obes 2021;28:533–9.
33. Dionisi-Vici M, Fantoni M, Botto R, et al. Distress, anxiety, depression and unmet needs in thyroid cancer survivors: a longitudinal study. Endocrine 2021;74: 603–10.
34. Li R, Li G, Wang Y, et al. Psychological Distress and Sleep Disturbance Throughout Thyroid Nodule Screening, Diagnosis, and Treatment. J Clin Endocrinol Metab 2021;106:e4221–30.
35. Wang S, Huang H, Wang L, et al. A Psychological Nursing Intervention for Patients With Thyroid Cancer on Psychological Distress and Quality of Life: A Randomized Clinical Trial. J Nerv Ment Dis 2020;208:533–9.
36. Husson O, Poort H, Sansom-Daly UM, et al. Psychological Distress and Illness Perceptions in Thyroid Cancer Survivors: Does Age Matter? J Adolesc Young Adult Oncol 2020;9:375–83.
37. Wang HL, McMillan SC, Vijayakumar N, et al. A Behavioral Physical Activity Intervention to Manage Moderate and Severe Fatigue Among Head and Neck Cancer Patients-Pre-efficacy Study in the National Institutes of Health ORBIT Model. Cancer Nurs 2019;42:E1–14.
38. Wang Y, Fan S, Wang H, et al. Pictorial Representation of Illness and Self Measure-Revised 2 (PRISM-R2): an effective tool to assess perceived burden of thyroid cancer in mainland China. Support Care Cancer 2018;26:3267–75.
39. Roerink SH, de Ridder M, Prins J, et al. High level of distress in long-term survivors of thyroid carcinoma: results of rapid screening using the distress thermometer. Acta Oncol 2013;52:128–37.
40. Papaleontiou M, Zebrack B, Reyes-Gastelum D, et al. Physician management of thyroid cancer patients' worry. J Cancer Surviv 2020;15(3):418–26.
41. Doubleday AR, Saucke MC, Bates MF, et al. Patient-surgeon decision-making about treatment for very low-risk thyroid cancer. Trends Cancer Res 2019;14: 79–89.
42. Pitt SC, Saucke MC, Roman BR, et al. The Influence of Emotions on Treatment Decisions About Low-Risk Thyroid Cancer: A Qualitative Study. Thyroid 2021; 31:1800–7.
43. Chen MM, Hughes TM, Dossett LA, et al. Peace of Mind: A Role in Unnecessary Care? J Clin Oncol 2022;40(5):433–7.
44. Loewenstein G, Weber EU, Hsee CK, et al. Risks as Feelings. Psychol Bull 2001; 127:267–86.
45. Hemmerich JA, Elstein AS, Schwarze ML, et al. Risk as feelings in the effect of patient outcomes on physicians' future treatment decisions: a randomized trial and manipulation validation. Social Sci Med (1982) 2012;75:367–76.
46. <Tversky_Kahneman_1974_Science_Judgement under Uncertaintly-Heuristics & Biases.pdf>.

47. Randle RW, Bushman N, Orne J, et al. Papillary thyroid cancer: The good and the bad of the "good cancer". Thyroid 2017;27(7):902–7.
48. Easley JMB, Robinson L. Its the "Good" Cancer, So Who Cares? Percieved Lack of Support_Among Young Thyroid Cancer Survivors. Oncol Nurs Forum 2013; 40:596–600.
49. Haymart MR. Association of the Word Cancer With Thyroid Cancer Treatment Decisions-A Rose by Any Other Name. JAMA Otolaryngol Head Neck Surg 2018;144:896.
50. Bilimoria KY, Bentrem DJ, Linn JG, et al. Utilization of total thyroidectomy for papillary thyroid cancer in the United States. Surgery 2007;142:906–13 [discussion: 13.e1-2].
51. Haymart MR, Banerjee M, Stewart AK, et al. Use of radioactive iodine for thyroid cancer. JAMA 2011;306:721–8.
52. Ware JE Jr, Sherbourne CD. The MOS 36-item short-form health survey (SF-36): I. Conceptual framework and item selection. Med Care 1992;473–83.
53. Cella D, Choi SW, Condon DM, et al. PROMIS® adult health profiles: efficient short-form measures of seven health domains. Value Health 2019;22:537–44.
54. Goswami S, Mongelli M, Peipert BJ, et al. Benchmarking health-related quality of life in thyroid cancer versus other cancers and United States normative data. Surgery 2018;164:986–92.
55. Watt T, Bjorner JB, Groenvold M, et al. Establishing construct validity for the thyroid-specific patient reported outcome measure (ThyPRO): an initial examination. Qual Life Res 2009;18:483–96.
56. Husson O, Haak HR, Mols F, et al. Development of a disease-specific health-related quality of life questionnaire (THYCA-QoL) for thyroid cancer survivors. Acta Oncologica 2013;52:447–54.
57. Jacobson BH, Johnson A, Grywalski C, et al. The voice handicap index (VHI) development and validation. Am J Speech-Language Pathol 1997;6:66–70.
58. Torrance GW. Utility approach to measuring health-related quality of life. J chronic Dis 1987;40:593–600.
59. Esnaola NF, Cantor SB, Sherman SI, et al. Optimal treatment strategy in patients with papillary thyroid cancer: a decision analysis. Surgery 2001;130:921–30.
60. Kebebew E, Duh QY, Clark OH. Total thyroidectomy or thyroid lobectomy in patients with low-risk differentiated thyroid cancer: surgical decision analysis of a controversy using a mathematical model. World J Surg 2000;24:1295–302.
61. Sejean K, Calmus S, Durand-Zaleski I, et al. Surgery versus medical follow-up in patients with asymptomatic primary hyperparathyroidism: a decision analysis. Eur J Endocrinol 2005;153:915–27.
62. McCabe C, Edlin R, Meads D, et al. Constructing indirect utility models: some observations on the principles and practice of mapping to obtain health state utilities. Pharmacoeconomics 2013;31:635–41.
63. Lubitz CC, De Gregorio L, Fingeret AL, et al. Measurement and Variation in Estimation of Quality of Life Effects of Patients Undergoing Treatment for Papillary Thyroid Carcinoma. Thyroid 2017;27:197–206.
64. Arora A, Swords C, Garas G, et al. The perception of scar cosmesis following thyroid and parathyroid surgery: a prospective cohort study. Int J Surg 2016; 25:38–43.
65. Hogikyan ND, Wodchis WP, Terrell JE, et al. Voice-related quality of life (V-RQOL) following type I thyroplasty for unilateral vocal fold paralysis. J Voice 2000;14:378–86.

66. Spector BC, Netterville JL, Billante C, et al. Quality-of-life assessment in patients with unilateral vocal cord paralysis. Otolaryngol Head Neck Surg 2001;125: 176–82.
67. Pei Y-C, Fang T-J, Hsin L-J, et al. Early hyaluronate injection improves quality of life but not neural recovery in unilateral vocal fold paralysis: an open-label randomized controlled study. Restorative Neurol Neurosci 2015;33:121–30.
68. Kumar V, Malhotra V, Sinha V. Evaluation of Individual Quality of Life (QOL) Among Patients with Tracheostomy Using WHO-QOL BREF Questionnaire. Indian J Otolaryngol Head Neck Surg 2020;1–10.
69. Dispenza F, Dispenza C, Marchese D, et al. Treatment of bilateral vocal cord paralysis following permanent recurrent laryngeal nerve injury. Am J Otolaryngol 2012;33:285–8.
70. Özdemir S, Tuncer Ü, Tarkan Ö, et al. Carbon dioxide laser endoscopic posterior cordotomy technique for bilateral abductor vocal cord paralysis: a 15-year experience. JAMA Otolaryngol Head Neck Surg 2013;139:401–4.
71. Berzofsky CE, Amy L, Pitman MJ. Postoperative management of superior laryngeal nerve paralysis. In: Randolph GW, editor. The recurrent and superior laryngeal nerves. Springer - Switzerland: Springer; 2016. p. 301–8.
72. Lifante J-C, McGill J, Murry T, et al. A prospective, randomized trial of nerve monitoring of the external branch of the superior laryngeal nerve during thyroidectomy under local/regional anesthesia and IV sedation. Surgery 2009;146: 1167–73.
73. Krekeler BN, Wendt E, Macdonald C, et al. Patient-reported dysphagia after thyroidectomy: a qualitative study. JAMA Otolaryngol Head Neck Surg 2018;144: 342–8.
74. Büttner M, Musholt TJ, Singer S. Quality of life in patients with hypoparathyroidism receiving standard treatment: a systematic review. Endocrine 2017;58: 14–20.
75. Astor MC, Løvås K, Debowska A, et al. Epidemiology and health-related quality of life in hypoparathyroidism in Norway. J Clin Endocrinol Metab 2016;101: 3045–53.
76. Tabacco G, Tay Y-KD, Cusano NE, et al. Quality of life in hypoparathyroidism improves with rhPTH (1-84) throughout 8 years of therapy. J Clin Endocrinol Metab 2019;104:2748–56.
77. Mallick U, Harmer C, Yap B, et al. Ablation with low-dose radioiodine and thyrotropin alfa in thyroid cancer. N Engl J Med 2012;366:1674–85.
78. Mernagh P, Suebwongpat A, Silverberg J, et al. Cost-effectiveness of using recombinant human thyroid-stimulating hormone before radioiodine ablation for thyroid cancer: the Canadian perspective. Value Health 2010;13:180–7.
79. Nygaard B, Bastholt L, Bennedbaek FN, et al. A placebo-controlled, blinded and randomised study on the effects of recombinant human thyrotropin on quality of life in the treatment of thyroid cancer. Eur Thyroid J 2013;2:195–202.
80. Hyer S, Kong A, Pratt B, et al. Salivary gland toxicity after radioiodine therapy for thyroid cancer. Clin Oncol 2007;19:83–6.
81. Dingle IF, Mishoe AE, Nguyen SA, et al. Salivary morbidity and quality of life following radioactive iodine for well-differentiated thyroid cancer. Otolaryngol Head Neck Surg 2013;148:746–52.
82. Haugen BR, Alexander EK, Bible KC, et al. 2015 American Thyroid Association Management Guidelines for Adult Patients with Thyroid Nodules and Differentiated Thyroid Cancer: The American Thyroid Association Guidelines Task Force on Thyroid Nodules and Differentiated Thyroid Cancer. Thyroid 2016;26:1–133.

83. Crevenna R, Zettinig G, Keilani M, et al. Quality of life in patients with non-metastatic differentiated thyroid cancer under thyroxine supplementation therapy. Support Care Cancer 2003;11:597–603.
84. Miller KD, Nogueira L, Mariotto AB, et al. Cancer treatment and survivorship statistics, 2019. CA Cancer J Clin 2019;69:363–85.
85. Jacobsen PB, Rowland JH, Paskett ED, et al. Identification of Key Gaps in Cancer Survivorship Research: Findings From the American Society of Clinical Oncology Survey. J Oncol Pract 2016;12:190–3.
86. SEER Cancer Stat Facts: Thyroid Cancer. National Cancer Institute, 2021. 2022. Available at: https://seer.cancer.gov/statfacts/html/thyro.html. Accessed January 2, 2022.
87. McIntyre C, Jacques T, Palazzo F, et al. Quality of life in differentiated thyroid cancer. Int J Surg 2018;50:133–6.
88. Husson O, Haak HR, Buffart LM, et al. Health-related quality of life and disease specific symptoms in long-term thyroid cancer survivors: a study from the population-based PROFILES registry. Acta Oncol 2013;52:249–58.
89. Dagan T, Bedrin L, Horowitz Z, et al. Quality of life of well-differentiated thyroid carcinoma patients. J Laryngol Otol 2004;118:537–42.
90. Applewhite MK, James BC, Kaplan SP, et al. Quality of Life in Thyroid Cancer is Similar to That of Other Cancers with Worse Survival. World J Surg 2016;40:551–61.
91. Lee JI, Kim SH, Tan AH, et al. Decreased health-related quality of life in disease-free survivors of differentiated thyroid cancer in Korea. Health Qual Life Outcomes 2010;8:101.
92. Chow KY, Kurumety S, Helenowski IB, et al. Association between quality of life and patient-reported complications from surgery and radioiodine in early-stage thyroid cancer survivors: A matched-pair analysis. Surgery 2021;170:462–8.
93. Kurumety SK, Helenowski IB, Goswami S, et al. Post-thyroidectomy neck appearance and impact on quality of life in thyroid cancer survivors. Surgery 2019;165:1217–21.
94. Pelttari H, Sintonen H, Schalin-Jantti C, et al. Health-related quality of life in long-term follow-up of patients with cured TNM Stage I or II differentiated thyroid carcinoma. Clin Endocrinol (Oxf) 2009;70:493–7.
95. Wrenn SM, Wang TS, Toumi A, et al. Practice patterns for surgical management of low-risk papillary thyroid cancer from 2014 to 2019: A CESQIP analysis. Am J Surg 2021;221:448–54.
96. Wong KP, Mak KL, Wong CK, et al. Systematic review and meta-analysis on intra-operative neuro-monitoring in high-risk thyroidectomy. Int J Surg 2017;38:21–30.
97. Colombo C, De Leo S, Di Stefano M, et al. Total Thyroidectomy Versus Lobectomy for Thyroid Cancer: Single-Center Data and Literature Review. Ann Surg Oncol 2021;28:4334–44.
98. Diez JJ, Anda E, Sastre J, et al. Recovery of parathyroid function in patients with thyroid cancer treated by total thyroidectomy: An analysis of 685 patients with hypoparathyroidism at discharge of surgery. Endocrinol Diabetes Nutr (Engl Ed) 2021;68:398–407.
99. Banach R, Bartes B, Farnell K, et al. Results of the Thyroid Cancer Alliance international patient/survivor survey: Psychosocial/informational support needs, treatment side effects and international differences in care. Hormones (Athens) 2013;12:428–38.

100. Goswami S, Peipert BJ, Mongelli MN, et al. Clinical factors associated with worse quality-of-life scores in United States thyroid cancer survivors. Surgery 2019;166:69–74.
101. Buttner M, Hinz A, Singer S, et al. Quality of life of patients more than 1 year after surgery for thyroid cancer. Hormones (Athens) 2020;19:233–43.
102. Frey S, Figueres L, Pattou F, et al. Impact of Permanent Post-thyroidectomy Hypoparathyroidism on Self-evaluation of Quality of Life and Voice: Results From the National QoL-Hypopara Study. Ann Surg 2021;274:851–8.
103. Nickel B, Tan T, Cvejic E, et al. Health-related quality of life after diagnosis and treatment of differentiated thyroid cancer and association with type of surgical treatment. JAMA Otolaryngol Head Neck Surg 2019;145:231–8.
104. van Gerwen M, Cooke PV, Alpert N, et al. Patient-reported outcomes following total thyroidectomy and lobectomy in thyroid cancer survivors: an analysis of the PROFILES Registry data. Support Care Cancer 2022;30:687–93.
105. Bongers PJ, Greenberg CA, Hsiao R, et al. Differences in long-term quality of life between hemithyroidectomy and total thyroidectomy in patients treated for low-risk differentiated thyroid carcinoma. Surgery 2020;167:94–101.
106. Clement SC, Peeters RP, Ronckers CM, et al. Intermediate and long-term adverse effects of radioiodine therapy for differentiated thyroid carcinoma–a systematic review. Cancer Treat Rev 2015;41:925–34.
107. Taieb D, Sebag F, Cherenko M, et al. Quality of life changes and clinical outcomes in thyroid cancer patients undergoing radioiodine remnant ablation (RRA) with recombinant human TSH (rhTSH): a randomized controlled study. Clin Endocrinol (Oxf) 2009;71:115–23.
108. Chen W, Li J, Peng S, et al. Association of Total Thyroidectomy or Thyroid Lobectomy With the Quality of Life in Patients With Differentiated Thyroid Cancer With Low to Intermediate Risk of Recurrence. JAMA Surg 2022;157(3):200–9.
109. Choi Y, Lee JH, Kim YH, et al. Impact of postthyroidectomy scar on the quality of life of thyroid cancer patients. Ann Dermatol 2014;26:693–9.
110. Ramsey S, Blough D, Kirchhoff A, et al. Washington State cancer patients found to be at greater risk for bankruptcy than people without a cancer diagnosis. Health Aff (Millwood) 2013;32:1143–52.
111. Mongelli MN, Giri S, Peipert BJ, et al. Financial burden and quality of life among thyroid cancer survivors. Surgery 2020;167:631–7.
112. SEER*Explorer: An interactive website for SEER cancer statistics Surveillance Research Program, National Cancer Institute.
113. Roman BR, Brito JP, Saucke MC, et al. National Survey of Endocrinologists and Surgeons Regarding Active Surveillance for Low-Risk Papillary Thyroid Cancer. Endocr Pract 2021;27:1–7.
114. Jeon MJ, Lee Y-M, Sung T-Y, et al. Quality of life in patients with papillary thyroid microcarcinoma managed by active surveillance or lobectomy: a cross-sectional study. Thyroid 2019;29:956–62.
115. Hedman C, Djarv T, Strang P, et al. Determinants of long-term quality of life in patients with differentiated thyroid carcinoma - a population-based cohort study in Sweden. Acta Oncol 2016;55:365–9.
116. Ito Y, Miyauchi A, Inoue H, et al. An observational trial for papillary thyroid microcarcinoma in Japanese patients. World J Surg 2010;34:28–35.
117. Tuttle RM, Fagin JA, Minkowitz G, et al. Natural History and Tumor Volume Kinetics of Papillary Thyroid Cancers During Active Surveillance. JAMA Otolaryngol Head Neck Surg 2017;143:1015–20.

118. Molinaro E, Campopiano MC, Pieruzzi L, et al. Active Surveillance in Papillary Thyroid Microcarcinomas is Feasible and Safe: Experience at a Single Italian Center. J Clin Endocrinol Metab 2020;105.
119. Group W. Development of the World Health Organization WHOQOL-BREF quality of life assessment. Psychol Med 1998;28:551–8.
120. Gliklich RE, Glovsky RM, Montgomery WW. Validation of a voice outcome survey for unilateral vocal cord paralysis. Otolaryngol Head Neck Surg 1999;120: 153–8.
121. Belafsky PC, Postma GN, Koufman JA. Validity and reliability of the reflux symptom index (RSI). J voice 2002;16:274–7.
122. Finlay AY, Khan G. Dermatology Life Quality Index (DLQI)—a simple practical measure for routine clinical use. Clin Exp Dermatol 1994;19:210–6.
123. Watt T, Hegedus L, Groenvold M, et al. Validity and reliability of the novel thyroid-specific quality of life questionnaire, ThyPRO. Eur J Endocrinol 2010;162:161–7.
124. Herschbach P, Berg P, Dankert A, et al. Fear of progression in chronic diseases: psychometric properties of the Fear of Progression Questionnaire. J psychosomatic Res 2005;58:505–11.
125. Henson B, Inglehart M, Eisbruch A, et al. Preserved salivary output and xerostomia-related quality of life in head and neck cancer patients receiving parotid-sparing radiotherapy. Oral Oncol 2001;37:84–93.
126. Chen AY, Frankowski R, Bishop-Leone J, et al. The development and validation of a dysphagia-specific quality-of-life questionnaire for patients with head and neck cancer: the MD Anderson dysphagia inventory. Arch Otolaryngol Head Neck Surg 2001;127:870–6.
127. Hassan SJ, Weymuller EA. Assessment of quality of life in head and neck cancer patients. Head & neck 1993;15:485–96.
128. Herdman M, Gudex C, Lloyd A, et al. Development and preliminary testing of the new five-level version of EQ-5D (EQ-5D-5L). Qual Life Res 2011;20:1727–36.
129. Brazier JE, Roberts J. The estimation of a preference-based measure of health from the SF-12. Med Care 2004;851–9.
130. Torrance GW, Feeny DH, Furlong WJ, et al. Multiattribute utility function for a comprehensive health status classification system: Health Utilities Index Mark 2. Med Care 1996;702–22.
131. Feeny D, Furlong W, Torrance GW, et al. Multiattribute and single-attribute utility functions for the health utilities index mark 3 system. Med Care 2002;40:113–28.

Use of Patient-Reported Outcomes for Assessing Diabetes Outcomes

Hyon Kim, MD[1,*], Kunal Shah, MD[1,*], Christoph Buettner, MD, PhD*

KEYWORDS

• Diabetes • Patient-reported outcomes • Insulin • Pumps • CGMs

KEY POINTS

- Patient-reported outcome (PRO) instruments are standardized questionnaires that directly assess the impact of a therapy or condition on the patient's perception of their overall health, treatment satisfaction, symptoms, and quality of life.
- PRO tools can evaluate patient-relevant factors that reduce medication or dietary adherence or reveal unintended treatment effects that would have otherwise not been captured by objective clinical measures.
- Improvement in clinical outcomes does not always correlate with improvement in PROs.
- There is no clear consensus on which PRO concepts or domains should be routinely included in diabetes studies, although a combination of tools should be used to comprehensively evaluate treatment effects.

INTRODUCTION

Diabetes is a complex chronic condition that currently affects approximately 34.2 million individuals in the United States alone.[1] The treatment of diabetes involves a multimodal approach focusing on diet, physical activity, weight management, and pharmacotherapy.[2–4] Living with diabetes can be particularly challenging for patients as this condition primarily requires self-management, such as frequent monitoring of glucose, daily attention to diet and exercise, and medication adherence. Therefore, it is critical to understand the patient's experience and identify barriers to care using standardized assessment tools to optimize the multidimensional management of diabetes.

Department of Medicine, Division of Endocrinology, Metabolism and Nutrition Rutgers, The State University of New Jersey, One Robert Wood Johnson Place, Medical Education Boulevard, 384, New Brunswick, NJ 08901, USA
[1] These authors contributed equally to this work.
* Corresponding authors.
E-mail addresses: hyonkim@rwjms.rutgers.edu (H.K.); shahk5@rwjms.rutgers.edu (K.S.); cb1116@rwjms.rutgers.edu (C.B.)

Endocrinol Metab Clin N Am 51 (2022) 781–793
https://doi.org/10.1016/j.ecl.2022.05.001

endo.theclinics.com

Patient-reported outcomes (PROs) refer to outcomes reported by the patient who experiences them first-hand. PROs are commonly assessed through questionnaires, called PRO instruments or PRO measures (PROMs), which offer a direct and systematic way to assess a patient's perception of their overall physical and mental well-being, disease symptoms, treatment side effects, and health-related quality of life (HR-QoL).[5,6] These assessments can be one-dimensional or multidimensional and can take less than 5 min to longer than 30 min to complete.[7] Although diabetes control is often evaluated by objective and measurable outcomes such as the hemoglobin A1c levels, PROs offer unique insights into the patient's experience with the treatment and may reveal unintended outcomes that would have otherwise not been captured.

Diabetes-specific PRO instruments can be used for targeted evaluation of diabetes self-management, including assessment of treatment satisfaction, distress related to dietary restriction or medication monitoring, emotional or social burdens related to diabetes treatment, and fear of hypoglycemia or diabetes complications.[7] One of the first diabetes-specific PRO tools was the diabetes quality-of-life (DQOL) scale which was developed for the Diabetes Control and Complications Trial.[8] DQOL assesses domains including satisfaction with diabetes treatment, impact of diabetes on activities of daily living such as driving or social relationships, concerns regarding the effect of diabetes on work and school, and concerns regarding complications of diabetes.[8] Several diabetes-specific PRO tools have since been developed, although there are currently no standardized approaches for using PROs in clinical trials of diabetes.[6] In this review, we provide a brief overview of how PRO instruments have been used to evaluate different modalities and complications of diabetes treatment and the valuable insights provided by the PROs for patient-centered diabetes management.

MEDICATIONS

Medication adherence is a key component of diabetes management, although reported adherence rates are overall poor, ranging from 36% to 93% for oral medications and 62% to 64% for insulin treatment in patients with type 2 diabetes.[9] Factors that could potentially reduce medication adherence include intensive regimens with multiple medications, route of administration (oral vs injection), psychosocial barriers such as depression and side effects such as hypoglycemia and weight gain. PRO instruments provide a standardized means to evaluate these patient-relevant factors or unintended outcomes of treatment.

There are currently no established recommendations for which core concepts or domains should be included in PRO instruments used in diabetes trials.[6] A recent review that evaluated PROs used in phase 3 clinical trials of the newer incretin-based therapies and Sodium Glucose Cotransporter-2 (SGLT2) inhibitors categorized the domains that were commonly examined as follows[1]: diabetes symptoms,[2] HR-QoL,[3] psychological well-being,[4] treatment/health satisfaction, and[5] impact of medication on weight.[5] It is important to consider multiple domains to provide a comprehensive assessment of a particular treatment. Depression is perhaps one of the most important domains to evaluate as diabetes can increase the risk of depression by twofold, and depressive symptoms are more frequently noted using patient-reported questionnaires as opposed to standardized interviews.[10] Studies have also shown an association between depression and poor adherence to therapy, which can lead to adverse outcomes.[11]

The Rimonabant in Obesity (RIO) trials on the use of the selective cannabinoid type 1 receptor antagonist rimonabant in overweight or obese patients with or without diabetes highlighted the need to assess whether a particular treatment could potentially worsen depression which up to then had not been routinely assessed in diabetes drug trials.[12] In the RIO-Diabetes trial, physical functioning scores improved in the rimonabant group as assessed by the Short Form 36 health survey questionnaire and the impact of weight on quality of life (IWQoL-Lite) PRO.[13] However, the Hospital Anxiety and Depression (HAD) scale showed a trend toward increased anxiety and depression in the treatment group. Patients on rimonabant were 2.5 times more likely to discontinue the drug due to depressive mood disorders.[12] Of note, the HAD scale did not specifically evaluate suicidal tendencies. Nevertheless, the food & drug administration (FDA) eventually did not approve rimonabant because of the evidence of a higher risk of suicide attempts or ideation in the treatment group,[14,15] illustrating that PROs can be highly valuable in identifying unexpected side effects.

The above example also underscores that the choice of PRO instruments is key to capturing unanticipated adverse events of diabetes drugs, and it may be best to choose a variety of PRO instruments to cover multiple domains. The choice of which PRO instrument(s) should be selected for a particular study depends on the specific clinical question being evaluated and the overall study design (eg, duration of follow-up, patient population).[16,17] One of the most commonly used PRO instruments that is recommended by the World Health Organization and the International Diabetes Federation is the Diabetes Treatment Satisfaction Questionnaire (DTSQ) and the change version, which is an updated version that allows patients to evaluate their current treatment in comparison to their previous treatment.[5,18,19] It has been translated into many languages and consists of only eight questions that are quick and easy to complete, which allows for its widespread use.[20] The DTSQ focuses on patient satisfaction with the treatment, the perceived convenience or flexibility of the treatment, and the ability of the patients to understand diabetes and their willingness to continue the current treatment or to recommend it to others. In addition, the frequency of hyper-and hypoglycemic episodes are also included in this questionnaire.[18]

The DTSQ has been used in several studies on glucagon-like peptide-1 (GLP-1) agonists, insulin, and SGLT2 inhibitors. It was used in the Assessment of Weekly Administration of Dulaglutide in Diabetes (AWARD)-1 and AWARD-3 trials which assessed dulaglutide versus placebo or exenatide and dulaglutide versus metformin, respectively, and showed that despite the inclusion of injectable therapy and gastrointestinal side effects, treatment satisfaction increased in the dulaglutide-treated group.[21] In the Semaglutide Unabated Sustainability in Treatment of Type 2 Diabetes 2 and 4 trials that assessed semaglutide versus sitagliptin and semaglutide versus glargine, respectively, the DTSQ showed that treatment satisfaction with semaglutide increased in spite of gastrointestinal side effects.[22] In the Liraglutide Effect and Action in Diabetes-6 trial that compared once-daily liraglutide versus twice-daily exenatide as add-on therapy to metformin and/or sulfonylurea therapy, the DTSQ score increased significantly in the liraglutide treatment group compared with exenatide due to higher scores in all the DTSQ items listed above, except for satisfaction with the understanding of diabetes.[23] In patients with type 1 diabetes, the DTSQ has also been used to show greater treatment satisfaction with glargine plus lispro insulin regimens over neutral protamine hagedorn (NPH) with unmodified human insulin.[24]

It is important to include diabetes-specific PRO tools in studies to assess the effects of diabetes medications as generic tools may not capture the unique outcomes related to diabetes. For example, the generic EuroQol-5 Dimension (EQ-5D) questionnaire did not elucidate differences between patients on maximally tolerated metformin and sulfonylurea therapy who were assigned to biphasic insulin, prandial insulin, or basal insulin daily in the treat-to-target in type 2 diabetes trial.[25,26]

However, the diabetes-specific Insulin Treatment Satisfaction Questionnaire (ITSQ) that evaluates the impact of insulin therapy on inconvenience of treatment, glycemic control, and lifestyle flexibility, showed the differences in treatment satisfaction between the groups.[25] Specifically, it showed that patients on prandial insulin regimens and those who experienced weight gain and hypoglycemia had significantly lower treatment satisfaction.

Although treatment satisfaction can impact the quality of life, the latter is not directly measured by DTSQ and ITSQ. On the other hand, the Audit of Diabetes-Dependent Quality of Life (ADDQoL) allows patients to rate the impact of diabetes on a particular domain such as “freedom to eat as I wish,” “unwanted dependence on others,” or “ease of traveling” and also evaluates the importance of that domain in their overall quality of life.[19] The Treatment Impact Measure for Diabetes is an example of a PRO that addresses multiple domains in addition to treatment satisfaction, such as quality of life, psychological health, and compliance.[27] This tool addresses concerns related to treatment burden including correct timing of medication, daily activities such as meal planning, and diabetes management such as the impact of the medication on episodes of hypoglycemia or hyperglycemia. Furthermore, overall compliance such as missing dosages and psychological health such as feelings of anger, depression, or worry related to complications of diabetes are also evaluated by this questionnaire.

Improvements in clinical outcomes may not always correlate with improved treatment satisfaction or other PROMs. For example, when dapagliflozin was added to metformin and sulfonylurea therapy in patients with poorly controlled diabetes (A1c >7%), there were significant improvements in hemoglobin A1c and weight loss compared with placebo.[28] However, this was not associated with increased treatment satisfaction as the DTSQ scores were not significantly different between treatment groups or from baseline. IWQoL-Lite, a PRO tool commonly used to assess the impact of weight on different domains such as physical function and self-esteem, was also not significantly different.[29] This discrepancy between patient treatment satisfaction and clinically objective outcomes illustrates that PROs can complement the assessment of objective, testing-based disease-specific outcomes.

DEVICES

Devices are crucial in diabetes care as they have significantly improved the patient experience in all aspects, from the administration of insulin to continuous glucose monitoring (CGM). PROs are extremely important in this context as satisfaction with a device can increase compliance and promote greater usage.

DEVICES: INSULIN PENS VERSUS SYRINGES

Currently, diabetes patients administer insulin using pens or vials and syringes.[30] The PRO assessment for these devices includes quality of life, confidence (device was used correctly), convenience (ease of use), acceptability (how many accepted using the device), and needle fear/pain. These assessments are vital for practitioners as they can assist in identifying the device that can best improve compliance and satisfaction.

Several studies have used PRO tools to confirm that insulin pens provide higher QoL over syringe applications and prove to be easier to use in part due to lower needle fear scores.[31,32] This was because of needles being less visible in pens and overall being sharper and thinner, leading to less pain with use.[32] Furthermore, 35% of patients anticipated pain from insulin management, and needle fear was even higher in patients who were unwilling to start insulin therapy,[33] which underscores the utility of these tools.

DEVICES: CONTINUOUS GLUCOSE MONITORS

The advent of CGMs has had a significant impact on the patient experience by improving confidence and control in diabetes patients and decreasing emotional stress and fear of hypoglycemia.[34] Several questionnaires have been used in studies to determine how CGMs affect PROs.[35,36]

Three scales that have been validated are Problem Areas in Diabetes (PAID)-5, Hypoglycemia Fear Survey-Worries (HFS-W), and confidence in diabetes self-care (CIDS) (**Table 1**). The PAID-5 questionnaire was developed specifically for recognizing diabetes-associated emotional distress, whereas the HFS-W was developed to determine the impact of an intervention on the concerns regarding hypoglycemia. The CIDS scale evaluates PROs related to self-confidence in diabetes management.[37–39]

All three assessments use a 5-point Likert scale and are widely used as they are short and easy to understand. One study that used all three assessments determined that CGMs overall decrease emotional distress and worry over hypoglycemia and increase self-confidence.[36]

However, there are some negative PROs associated with CGMs, including information overload, alarm fatigue, and physical discomfort. Patients who described themselves as being more comfortable with technology had greater treatment satisfaction with CGMs compared with those who did not feel comfortable with technology.[40] In addition, one study assessed the causal factors of the unwillingness to use a CGM and found that discomfort from use and alarm fatigue were the major reasons.[41]

Although CGMs may offer significant benefits to diabetes patients, assessment of PROs has shown that CGMs are not universally popular and appropriate patient selection is important.

DEVICES: INSULIN PUMPS

Insulin pumps provide an automated delivery system of insulin and have been shown to reduce hemoglobin A1c when compared with daily injections.[42] Traditional insulin pumps were developed to provide a continuous infusion of insulin that was managed by manual patient input. PROs for insulin pumps are important to consider as QoL measures such as convenience, satisfaction, physical discomfort, and ease of use can affect compliance with these devices.

The Insulin Delivery System Rating Questionnaire (IDSRQ) is used to measure PROs specifically dealing with the methods of insulin delivery.[43] It consists of a subscale

Table 1
Problem Areas in Diabetes-5, Hypoglycemia Fear Survey-Worries, confidence in diabetes self-care are three scales used in determining continuous glucose monitor patient-reported outcomes

Survey	PRO Measured	Length	Scale
Problem Areas in Diabetes	Emotional distress in diabetes	5 items	Likert 5-point
Hypoglycemia Fear Survey-Worries	Anticipatory hypoglycemia fear	18 items	Likert 5-point
Confidence in diabetes self-care	Confidence in managing diabetes	20 items	Likert 5-point

Adapted from Nefs G, Bazelmans E, Marsman D, Snellen N, Tack CJ, de Galan BE. RT-CGM in adults with type 1 diabetes improves both glycaemic and patient-reported outcomes, but independent of each other. Diabetes Res Clin Pract. 2019;158:107910.

directly related to the method of delivery and quality of life measures such as satisfaction, level of interference with daily living and pain/discomfort, and a more general subscale that indirectly assesses insulin pumps such as psychological well-being associated with diabetes.

One study used IDSRQ to measure PROs for insulin pumps along with EQ-5D that uses a visual analog scale to assess similar QOL measures as IDSRQ but also incorporates cost-effectiveness and the Diabetes Symptom Checklist-Revised (DSC-R) which assesses symptoms associated with diabetes such as hyperglycemia, hypoglycemia, and psychological well-being.[44] Patients who used insulin pumps overall scored better in terms of reduction of symptoms as compared with patients using multiple daily injections (MDIs). Specifically, as assessed by the DSC-R, patients had improved fatigue scores. Anticipatory hypoglycemia fear and overall psychological well-being were significantly higher as per EQ-5D, and satisfaction was scored better according to IDSRQ. There was a strong preference for the pump over MDI and there was no significant increase in interference in daily life with the former.

In addition, QoL was improved in patients using pumps over an MDI regimen because of a reduction in A1c and variations in blood glucose levels provided by the insulin pumps. It was hypothesized that significant glucose variability affects mood and increases fear of hypoglycemia.[45] The IDRSQ was used to validate this hypothesis and indeed identified a link between the reduction in A1c and glucose variability with improved QoL in patients who were initiated on insulin pumps.[46]

DEVICES: HYBRID CLOSED-LOOP SYSTEMS

Hybrid closed-loop insulin pumps are connected to CGMs that provide real-time feedback and automatically adjust insulin infusion rates.

The two most commonly used hybrid closed-loop systems currently available are the Tandem T-Slim X2 with Control-IQ and the Medtronic MiniMed Series with Auto Mode. PROs can be used to help select patients for these devices and assess specific QOL measures such as sleep awakenings/quality, efficiency of use/connectivity to CGM, and trust in the system.

The Tandem T-Slim X2 system can significantly improve time in range, an important factor in glucose control, as compared with traditional insulin pump systems.[47] The system scored extremely high in treatment satisfaction which was attributed to strong sensor accuracy when connecting to the Dexcom CGM system, improved diabetes control, improved sleep quality because of decreased anticipatory fear of hypoglycemia and effective CGM connectivity.[48]

The Medtronic MiniMed 670G system can also provide improved glycemic control for some patients compared with non-hybrid closed-loop pump systems.[49] Patients reported high treatment satisfaction with this system, which was again related to decreased anticipatory fear of hypoglycemia and improved diabetes control. However, unlike the Tandem T-Slim system, one study noted frustration regarding the ease of use with Auto Mode and a significant cohort reported decreased satisfaction owing to connectivity difficulties with Auto Mode and Guardian sensor.[50] This issue had been noted in several other studies as well, with one study reporting 19% of participants discontinued the Medtronic 670G system due to technical difficulties.[51]

Overall, the importance of implementing PROs cannot be understated as they can help promote greater treatment satisfaction for diabetes patients and help normalize new technologies.

DIET

A healthy diet is the foundation of diabetes management as it can help maintain appropriate blood sugar levels. PROs provide insights into the perceived barriers and identify tools that may help patients accept dietary recommendations for diabetes such as carbohydrate and caloric restriction.[52]

The PROs that are most important to consider are tolerability, patient satisfaction, and feasibility (cost, taste, access to food). Targeting these may help providers understand how best to improve a patient's compliance with a prescribed diet.

In general, a low carbohydrate diet is the preferred diabetes compliant regimen, as it lowers A1c and improves glycemic control. Modifying one's lifestyle can be difficult as many persons are resistant to changing old habits, especially at older ages, and diabetes compliant regimens are often construed as rigid and constraining.[53,54] There is evidence of comparable or even better adherence to low-carbohydrate diets than other calorically similar dietary regimens if the patients are appropriately counseled by the clinicians.[54] Patients on low-carbohydrate diets may also experience lower appetite when compared with other diets. This is an important PRO to acknowledge not only for diabetes but also for weight loss. Unfortunately, the data behind this are limited to only short-term studies.[55]

Carbohydrate counting is an important tool that can be used to improve glycemic control in patients with both type 1 and type 2 diabetes,[56] although psychosocial measures must be taken into account in the case of adolescent patients. The EQ-5D was used for QoL evaluation and showed improvement in subjective well-being after receiving carbohydrate counting training. Part of this was linked to the glycemic benefits that were seen by the carb counting cohort. In the dose adjustment for normal eating (DAFNE) study, however, the ADDQoL showed no clinically meaningful improvement in QoL when comparing advanced carb counting versus a control group in adolescents with type 1 diabetes.[57]

A newly popular dietary strategy for diabetes is intermittent fasting, which can improve insulin resistance and may be as effective as a caloric restriction diet for reducing hemoglobin A1c.[58,59] However, some studies have shown that intermittent fasting may be less feasible and provide less adherence when compared with daily caloric restriction. One long-term study showed a self-reported discontinuation rate of intermittent fasting in 71% of the participants as opposed to 32.5% in patients on continuous caloric restriction after 50 weeks.[60] Therefore, although intermittent fasting is a modality that can be implemented for improving diabetes control, adherence must be considered before starting this regimen.

The Mediterranean diet is another popular option that has shown some benefit in improving glycemic control in diabetes.[61] Adherence to the diet is the most important PRO and is associated with greater diabetes treatment satisfaction.[62] Diabetes-specific surveys such as the DTSQ and ADDQoL were used to show that patients on the Mediterranean diet were more likely to recommend this treatment to others, had improved self-confidence relating to diabetes management, and scored highly on "freedom to drink" and "freedom to eat" which were perceptions based on ease of access and reduction of limitations of what patients could eat.[63]

Adherence to any diet, including intermittent fasting and the Mediterranean diet, has a strong impact on QoL and is often associated with patient motivation.[63,64] Unfortunately, many studies assessing PROs on dietary impact and adherence are short term. Longer term studies are needed as adherence may be strong in the short term but wane with time.[60,65]

SUMMARY

PROs provide invaluable insights into the impact of diabetes and its different treatment modalities on a patient's overall health status and QoL. PRO tools can be used to identify barriers to treatment adherence and reveal patient preferences for one treatment modality over another, such as insulin pen versus syringe delivery. They can also capture patient-relevant factors such as depression, which could otherwise not be discerned using objective, testing-based outcome measurements. PRO instruments can also assess patients' concerns regarding diabetes technology such as CGMs and hybrid closed-loop insulin pumps. They can evaluate factors that impact compliance with these devices, including convenience, reduction in anticipatory fear of hypoglycemia, or interference with daily life and physical discomfort. PROs can also guide counseling about diet and exercise. Multiple studies have evaluated adherence to diets and explored PROs such as freedom and convenience that may impact adherence.

There has been a growing interest in the use of PRO instruments in diabetes clinical trials despite the lack of a standard approach.[6] A clear consensus still needs to emerge on the key concepts and domains that should be routinely addressed by PRO instruments, as well as the optimal time window for using these assessments to capture the effects of a particular intervention. This will likely be specific to the interventions that are being evaluated. Using multiple PROMs may provide a comprehensive assessment of the impact of therapy.[66] Using PROs as primary outcomes instead of secondary or exploratory outcomes in clinical studies with larger populations and longer duration of follow-up may further elucidate treatment benefits or adverse events.[5] There are several areas of interest that need long-term follow-up with PROMs, such as adherence to diet which can wane over time. Another potential area for further study is the use of PROMs in clinical practice settings.[67] PROMs can take anywhere from 5 min to greater than 30 min to complete.[5,7] Therefore, use of PROMs that can be reasonably incorporated into a clinical visit to provide specific feedback about patient experiences may identify barriers to treatment adherence in real-time that can be immediately addressed. However, whether this translates into meaningful improvements in clinical outcomes remains to be examined.[67]

CLINICS CARE POINTS

- GLP-1 agonists, specifically dulaglutide, semaglutide, and liraglutide, improve patient satisfaction.
- Diabetes medications that increase weight gain and/or increase hypoglycemia, such as insulin, should be avoided if alternatives are available.
- Insulin therapy using pens can help reduce needle fear and increase adherence.
- Patient selection is important for continuous glucose monitor use as patients who are more technologically savvy may benefit more.
- Insulin pumps should be encouraged for patients with significant glucose variability. Hybrid closed-loop insulin pumps may provide an even more benefit for patients.
- Dietary changes for diabetes care should be focused on adherence and counseling.
- The Mediterranean diet may be an advantageous option for diabetes patients because of improved adherence and satisfaction.

DISCLOSURE

The authors have no commercial or financial conflicts of interest.

REFERENCES

1. CDC. National diabetes statistics report, 2020. Atlanta (GA): Centers for Disease Control and Prevention, U.S. Dept of Health and Human Services; 2020.
2. American Diabetes Association Professional Practice C, American Diabetes Association Professional Practice C, Draznin B, Aroda VR, Bakris G, et al. 9. Pharmacologic Approaches to Glycemic Treatment: Standards of Medical Care in Diabetes-2022. Diabetes Care 2022;45(Supplement_1):S125–43.
3. American Diabetes Association Professional Practice C, American Diabetes Association Professional Practice C, Draznin B, Aroda VR, Bakris G, et al. 8. Obesity and Weight Management for the Prevention and Treatment of Type 2 Diabetes: Standards of Medical Care in Diabetes-2022. Diabetes Care 2022; 45(Supplement_1):S113–24.
4. American Diabetes Association Professional Practice C, American Diabetes Association Professional Practice C, Draznin B, Aroda VR, Bakris G, et al. 5. Facilitating Behavior Change and Well-being to Improve Health Outcomes: Standards of Medical Care in Diabetes-2022. Diabetes Care 2022;45(Supplement_1): S60–82.
5. Reaney M, Elash CA, Litcher-Kelly L. Patient Reported Outcomes (PROs) used in recent Phase 3 trials for Type 2 Diabetes: A review of concepts assessed by these PROs and factors to consider when choosing a PRO for future trials. Diabetes Res Clin Pract 2016;116:54–67.
6. Marrero DG, Hilliard ME, Maahs DM, et al. Using patient reported outcomes in diabetes research and practice: Recommendations from a national workshop. Diabetes Res Clin Pract 2019;153:23–9.
7. El Achhab Y, Nejjari C, Chikri M, et al. Disease-specific health-related quality of life instruments among adults diabetic: A systematic review. Diabetes Res Clin Pract 2008;80(2):171–84.
8. Reliability and validity of a diabetes quality-of-life measure for the diabetes control and complications trial (DCCT). The DCCT Research Group. Diabetes Care 1988;11(9):725–32.
9. Cramer JA. A systematic review of adherence with medications for diabetes. Diabetes Care 2004;27(5):1218–24.
10. Anderson RJ, Freedland KE, Clouse RE, et al. The prevalence of comorbid depression in adults with diabetes: a meta-analysis. Diabetes Care 2001;24(6): 1069–78.
11. Lin EH, Katon W, Von Korff M, et al. Relationship of depression and diabetes self-care, medication adherence, and preventive care. Diabetes Care 2004;27(9): 2154–60.
12. Christensen R, Kristensen PK, Bartels EM, et al. Efficacy and safety of the weight-loss drug rimonabant: a meta-analysis of randomised trials. Lancet 2007; 370(9600):1706–13.
13. Scheen AJ, Finer N, Hollander P, et al. Efficacy and tolerability of rimonabant in overweight or obese patients with type 2 diabetes: a randomised controlled study. Lancet 2006;368(9548):1660–72.
14. Mitchell PB, Morris MJ. Depression and anxiety with rimonabant. Lancet 2007; 370(9600):1671–2.

15. Sam AH, Salem V, Ghatei MA. Rimonabant: From RIO to Ban. J Obes 2011;2011: 432607.
16. Calvert M, Blazeby J, Altman DG, et al. Reporting of patient-reported outcomes in randomized trials: the CONSORT PRO extension. JAMA 2013;309(8):814–22.
17. Calvert M, Kyte D, Mercieca-Bebber R, et al. Guidelines for Inclusion of Patient-Reported Outcomes in Clinical Trial Protocols: The SPIRIT-PRO Extension. JAMA 2018;319(5):483–94.
18. Davies M, Speight J. Patient-reported outcomes in trials of incretin-based therapies in patients with type 2 diabetes mellitus. Diabetes Obes Metab 2012;14(10): 882–92.
19. Bradley C, Speight J. Patient perceptions of diabetes and diabetes therapy: assessing quality of life. Diabetes Metab Res Rev 2002;18(Suppl 3):S64–9.
20. Saisho Y. Use of Diabetes Treatment Satisfaction Questionnaire in Diabetes Care: Importance of Patient-Reported Outcomes. Int J Environ Res Public Health 2018; 15(5):947.
21. Reaney M, Yu M, Lakshmanan M, et al. Treatment satisfaction in people with type 2 diabetes mellitus treated with once-weekly dulaglutide: data from the AWARD-1 and AWARD-3 clinical trials. Diabetes Obes Metab 2015;17(9):896–903.
22. Jendle J, Birkenfeld AL, Polonsky WH, et al. Improved treatment satisfaction in patients with type 2 diabetes treated with once-weekly semaglutide in the SUSTAIN trials. Diabetes Obes Metab 2019;21(10):2315–26.
23. Schmidt WE, Christiansen JS, Hammer M, et al. Patient-reported outcomes are superior in patients with Type 2 diabetes treated with liraglutide as compared with exenatide, when added to metformin, sulphonylurea or both: results from a randomized, open-label study. Diabet Med 2011;28(6):715–23.
24. Ashwell SG, Bradley C, Stephens JW, et al. Treatment satisfaction and quality of life with insulin glargine plus insulin lispro compared with NPH insulin plus unmodified human insulin in individuals with type 1 diabetes. Diabetes Care 2008;31(6):1112–7.
25. Farmer AJ, Oke J, Stevens R, et al. Differences in insulin treatment satisfaction following randomized addition of biphasic, prandial or basal insulin to oral therapy in type 2 diabetes. Diabetes Obes Metab 2011;13(12):1136–41.
26. Holman RR, Thorne KI, Farmer AJ, et al. Addition of biphasic, prandial, or basal insulin to oral therapy in type 2 diabetes. N Engl J Med 2007;357(17):1716–30.
27. Brod M, Hammer M, Christensen T, et al. Understanding and assessing the impact of treatment in diabetes: the Treatment-Related Impact Measures for Diabetes and Devices (TRIM-Diabetes and TRIM-Diabetes Device). Health Qual Life Outcomes 2009;7:83.
28. Matthaei S, Bowering K, Rohwedder K, et al. Dapagliflozin improves glycemic control and reduces body weight as add-on therapy to metformin plus sulfonylurea: a 24-week randomized, double-blind clinical trial. Diabetes Care 2015; 38(3):365–72.
29. Grandy S, Sternhufvud C, Ryden A, et al. Patient-reported outcomes among patients with type 2 diabetes mellitus treated with dapagliflozin in a triple-therapy regimen for 52 weeks. Diabetes Obes Metab 2016;18(3):306–9.
30. Molife C, Lee LJ, Shi L, et al. Assessment of patient-reported outcomes of insulin pen devices versus conventional vial and syringe. Diabetes Technol Ther 2009; 11(8):529–38.
31. Simmons JH, McFann KK, Brown AC, et al. Reliability of the diabetes fear of injecting and self-testing questionnaire in pediatric patients with type 1 diabetes. Diabetes care 2007;30(4):987–8.

32. Anderson BJ, Redondo MJ. What can we learn from patient-reported outcomes of insulin pen devices? J Diabetes Sci Technol 2011;5(6):1563–71.
33. Polonsky WH, Fisher L, Guzman S, et al. Psychological insulin resistance in patients with type 2 diabetes: the scope of the problem. Diabetes care 2005;28(10):2543–5.
34. Rubin RR, Peyrot M. Patient-reported outcomes and diabetes technology: a systematic review of the literature. Pediatr Endocrinol Rev PER. 2010;7:405–12.
35. van Beers CA, Kleijer SJ, Serné EH, et al. Design and rationale of the IN CONTROL trial: the effects of real-time continuous glucose monitoring on glycemia and quality of life in patients with type 1 diabetes mellitus and impaired awareness of hypoglycemia. BMC Endocr Disord 2015;15(1):1–9.
36. Nefs G, Bazelmans E, Marsman D, et al. RT-CGM in adults with type 1 diabetes improves both glycaemic and patient-reported outcomes, but independent of each other. Diabetes Res Clin Pract 2019;158:107910.
37. McGuire B, Morrison T, Hermanns N, et al. Short-form measures of diabetes-related emotional distress: the Problem Areas in Diabetes Scale (PAID)-5 and PAID-1. Diabetologia 2010;53(1):66–9.
38. Lam AYR, Xin X, Tan WB, et al. Psychometric validation of the Hypoglycemia Fear Survey-II (HFS-II) in Singapore. BMJ Open Diabetes Res Care 2017;5(1):e000329.
39. Van Der Ven NC, Weinger K, Yi J, et al. The confidence in diabetes self-care scale: psychometric properties of a new measure of diabetes-specific self-efficacy in Dutch and US patients with type 1 diabetes. Diabetes care 2003;26(3):713–8.
40. Anhalt H. Limitations of continuous glucose monitor usage. Diabetes Technol Ther 2016;18(3):115–7.
41. Ramchandani N, Arya S, Ten S, et al. Real-life utilization of real-time continuous glucose monitoring: the complete picture. J Diabetes Sci Technol 2011;5(4):860–70.
42. Reznik Y, Cohen O, Aronson R, et al. Insulin pump treatment compared with multiple daily injections for treatment of type 2 diabetes (OpT2mise): a randomised open-label controlled trial. Lancet 2014;384(9950):1265–72.
43. Peyrot M, Rubin RR. Validity and reliability of an instrument for assessing health-related quality of life and treatment preferences: the Insulin Delivery System Rating Questionnaire. Diabetes Care 2005;28(1):53–8.
44. Rubin RR, Peyrot M, Chen X, et al. Patient-reported outcomes from a 16-week open-label, multicenter study of insulin pump therapy in patients with type 2 diabetes mellitus. Diabetes Technol Ther 2010;12(11):901–6.
45. Cox DJ, McCall A, Kovatchev B, et al. Effects of blood glucose rate of changes on perceived mood and cognitive symptoms in insulin-treated type 2 diabetes. Diabetes Care 2007;30(8):2001–2.
46. Peyrot M, Rubin RR, Chen X, et al. Associations between improved glucose control and patient-reported outcomes after initiation of insulin pump therapy in patients with type 2 diabetes mellitus. Diabetes Technol Ther 2011;13(4):471–6.
47. Brown SA, Kovatchev BP, Raghinaru D, et al. Six-month randomized, multicenter trial of closed-loop control in type 1 diabetes. N Engl J Med 2019;381(18):1707–17.
48. Pinsker JE, Müller L, Constantin A, et al. Real-world patient-reported outcomes and glycemic results with initiation of control-IQ technology. Diabetes Technol Ther 2021;23(2):120–7.

49. Duffus SH, Ta'ani ZA, Slaughter JC, et al. Increased proportion of time in hybrid closed-loop "Auto Mode" is associated with improved glycaemic control for adolescent and young patients with adult type 1 diabetes using the MiniMed 670G insulin pump. Diabetes Obes Metab 2020;22(4):688–93.
50. DuBose SN, Bauza C, Verdejo A, et al. Real-World, Patient-Reported and Clinic Data from Individuals with Type 1 Diabetes Using the MiniMed 670G Hybrid Closed-Loop System. Diabetes Technol Ther 2021;23(12):791–8.
51. Goodwin G, Waldman G, Lyons J, et al. OR14-5 Challenges in implementing Hybrid Closed Loop Insulin Pump Therapy (medtronic 670g) In A'Real World'Clinical Setting. J Endocr Soc 2019;3(Supplement_1):OR14–5.
52. Kaplan RM, Hartwell SL, Wilson DK, et al. Effects of diet and exercise interventions on control and quality of life in non-insulin-dependent diabetes mellitus. J Gen Intern Med 1987;2(4):220–8.
53. Booth AO, Lowis C, Dean M, et al. Diet and physical activity in the self-management of type 2 diabetes: barriers and facilitators identified by patients and health professionals. Prim Health Care Res Dev 2013;14(3):293–306.
54. Feinman RD, Pogozelski WK, Astrup A, et al. Dietary carbohydrate restriction as the first approach in diabetes management: critical review and evidence base. Nutrition 2015;31(1):1–13.
55. Meng Y, Bai H, Wang S, et al. Efficacy of low carbohydrate diet for type 2 diabetes mellitus management: a systematic review and meta-analysis of randomized controlled trials. Diabetes Res Clin Pract 2017;131:124–31.
56. Souto DL, Rosado EL. Use of carb counting in the dietary treatment of diabetes mellitus. Nutricion Hospitalaria 2010;25(1):18–25.
57. Schmidt S, Schelde B, Nørgaard K. Effects of advanced carbohydrate counting in patients with type 1 diabetes: a systematic review. Diabetic Med 2014;31(8):886–96.
58. de Cabo R, Mattson MP. Effects of intermittent fasting on health, aging, and disease. N Engl J Med 2019;381(26):2541–51.
59. Borgundvaag E, Mak J, Kramer CK. Metabolic impact of intermittent fasting in patients with type 2 diabetes mellitus: a systematic review and meta-analysis of interventional studies. J Clin Endocrinol Metab 2021;106(3):902–11.
60. Pannen ST, Maldonado SG, Nonnenmacher T, et al. Adherence and Dietary Composition during Intermittent vs. Continuous Calorie Restriction: Follow-Up Data from a Randomized Controlled Trial in Adults with Overweight or Obesity. Nutrients 2021;13(4):1195.
61. Schröder H. Protective mechanisms of the Mediterranean diet in obesity and type 2 diabetes. J Nutr Biochem 2007;18(3):149–60.
62. Alcubierre N, Martinez-Alonso M, Valls J, et al. Relationship of the adherence to the Mediterranean diet with health-related quality of life and treatment satisfaction in patients with type 2 diabetes mellitus: a post-hoc analysis of a cross-sectional study. Health Qual Life Outcomes 2016;14(1):1–6.
63. Granado-Casas M, Martin M, Martinez-Alonso M, et al. The Mediterranean Diet is Associated with an Improved Quality of Life in Adults with Type 1 Diabetes. Nutrients 2020;12(1):131.
64. Arnason TG, Bowen MW, Mansell KD. Effects of intermittent fasting on health markers in those with type 2 diabetes: A pilot study. World J Diabetes 2017;8(4):154.
65. Alhassan S, Kim S, Bersamin A, et al. Dietary adherence and weight loss success among overweight women: results from the A TO Z weight loss study. Int J Obes 2008;32(6):985–91.

66. Bradley C, Eschwege E, de Pablos-Velasco P, et al. Predictors of Quality of Life and Other Patient-Reported Outcomes in the PANORAMA Multinational Study of People With Type 2 Diabetes. Diabetes Care 2018;41(2):267–76.
67. Skovlund SE, Lichtenberg TH, Hessler D, et al. Can the Routine Use of Patient-Reported Outcome Measures Improve the Delivery of Person-Centered Diabetes Care? A Review of Recent Developments and a Case Study. Curr Diab Rep 2019;19(9):84.

Physiology of the Weight-Reduced State and Its Impact on Weight Regain

Samar Hafida, MD[a,*], Caroline Apovian, MD, FTOS, DABOM[b]

KEYWORDS

• Obesity • Physiology of obesity • Weight-reduced state • Weight regain
• Bariatric surgery • Pharmacotherapy for obesity management

KEY POINTS

- Obesity is a chronic disease characterized by periods of remission (weight loss) and relapse (weight regain).
- Most individuals who lose weight are at risk for weight regain regardless of the weight loss intervention.
- The state of active weight loss differs from the weight-reduced state, where some metabolic adaptations persist for a considerable duration of time.
- Identifying factors associated with a higher risk of weight regain may allow clinicians to implement early interventions to improve weight loss outcomes.

INTRODUCTION

Obesity is a chronic disease characterized by increased energy intake to defend a dysregulated set point with periods of remission and relapses that result in a pathologic accumulation of adipose tissue resulting in increased morbidity and mortality. Obesity is similar to other chronic disease models such as diabetes, cancer, and cardiovascular disease, in that it has a long duration, slow progression, and periods of remission and relapses.[1] Globally, the prevalence of obesity has tripled since the mid-1970s, with nearly 2 billion adults and 340 million children and adolescents are either overweight or living with obesity.[2] Despite the rising prevalence, there has been an abundance of scientific breakthroughs, pharmacotherapies, behavioral interventions, technologies, and surgical options that have advanced the field of obesity

[a] Division of Endocrinology, Diabetes, Nutrition and Weight Management, 72 East, Concord Street C3 (Room 321 A), Collamore Building, Boston, MA 02118, USA; [b] Division of Endocrinology, Diabetes and Hypertension, Center for Weight Management and Wellness, Brigham and Women's Hospital, Harvard Medical School, 221 Longwood Avenue, Suite RFB-2, Brigham and Women's at 221 Longwood, Boston, MA 02115, USA
* Corresponding author.
E-mail address: Samar.hafida@bmc.org

Endocrinol Metab Clin N Am 51 (2022) 795–815
https://doi.org/10.1016/j.ecl.2022.06.002

medicine in the past two decades. Furthermore, it has been estimated that 42% of people living with obesity worldwide relentlessly conduct serious personal efforts to manage their weight using a variety of strategies every year.[3] This review will focus on the prevalence, explore the physiology of the weight-reduced state, describe potential mechanisms that oppose weight loss and facilitate weight regain, outline strategies to mitigate weight regain, and discuss patient-reported outcomes in the setting of weight regain.

PREVALENCE OF WEIGHT REGAIN

There is ample evidence that weight loss maintenance in individuals with obesity is difficult. The National Weight Control Registry,[4] established in 1993 to track and prospectively investigate characteristics of individuals with long-term weight loss maintenance, includes 10,000 members and is the largest of its kind. A 10-year observational study of 2886 individuals (78% female) who had lost at least 30 pounds in the first year revealed that more than 87% sustained 10% or more of their original weight loss after 10 years. Factors common among these individuals who continued to maintain a lower body weight were frequency of self-monitoring weight, maintaining a reduced-calorie diet, and larger initial weight loss.[5] On the other hand, the role physical activity (PA) plays in maintaining a weight loss is less evident. Although undoubtedly beneficial to many individuals who engage in regular high levels of PA, others may maintain weight loss with considerably lower levels of PA.[6] These differences among individuals who have maintained a weight-reduced state reflect the heterogeneous nature of factors that regulate body weight and the complex nature of interactions between environment and physiology.

A. *Weight regain after lifestyle intervention:* Clinical practice guidelines for the management of obesity recommend dietary modification, increased PA, and behavioral therapy as the foundation of weight management.[7] Implementation of a structured low-calorie diet and regular PA results in an average weight reduction of 8% to 10%,[8] which correlates with improvement in metabolic health. Most of the weight loss generated by lifestyle changes is derived from reducing caloric intake (80%), whereas PA contributes to approximately 20% of achieved weight loss.[8] Large-scale weight loss studies such as the Look AHEAD[9] and Diabetes Prevention Program (DPP)[10] have shown the ability of participants to achieve weight loss. However, weight maintenance and prevention of weight gain have remained challenging, particularly as sustaining the cardio metabolic benefits generated from these interventions is closely linked to maintaining a weight-reduced state. In the Look AHEAD trial, 68% of participants who received the intensive lifestyle intervention lost $\geq$ 5% of their body weight after 1 year, and 37.7% lost $\geq$ 10%. After a follow-up period of 8 years, 50.3% of individuals had lost $\geq$ 5% of their initial weight, whereas 26.9% lost 10% despite a high retention rate of $\geq$ 88% of participants who completed the 8-year follow-up period.[11] Another retrospective follow-up study evaluated weight loss maintenance in individuals with severe obesity enrolled in a 21-week weight loss camp where the average weight loss was 15% after the intervention. After 2–4 years, the average weight loss from baseline declined to 5.3%.[12]
B. *Weight regain after pharmacotherapy:* Pharmacotherapy for weight management with an FDA-approved medication is recommended for long-term management of obesity in individuals with a body mass index (BMI) of 30 kg/m^2 or 27 kg/m^2 (25 kg/m^2 in people of Asian descent) with one or more obesity-associated comorbidity such as type 2 diabetes, dyslipidemia, or hypertension.[7] A study of

Liraglutide 3.0 mg versus placebo[13] revealed that after 1 year, participants randomized to Liraglutide lost significantly more weight (−9.2% vs −3.5%) than placebo, and this remained significant after 3 years where weight was maintained at −6.1% of baseline weight in the Liraglutide group and −1.9% in the placebo group. In the STEP 4 study comparing once-weekly Semaglutide 2.4 mg versus placebo on weight loss maintenance, participants who were blindly switched to placebo after 20 weeks of receiving the Semaglutide regained most of their weight back after 68 weeks. Weight loss after the study period was −7.9% in the treatment group versus +6.9% P (<0.001) in the placebo group despite both receiving lifestyle treatment.[14] These findings support the critical role pharmacotherapy has in reducing rates of weight regain.

C. *Weight regain after metabolic (bariatric) surgery:* Metabolic surgery is the most effective intervention for obesity management. However, weight regain remains a significant challenge to individuals who undergo this procedure, potentially derailing its benefits.[15,16] There is no consensus on how to define weight regain. Some studies use excess weight loss (EWL), others use nadir weight, BMI, or any weight regain. Approximately 38% of individuals after laparoscopic adjustable gastric banding,[17] 27.8% after laparoscopic sleeve gastrectomy,[18] and 3.9% after roux-en Y gastric bypass[19] report weight regain. Furthermore, insufficient weight loss, defined as losing less than 50% of excess weight at 18 months post-surgery,[20] is the most common cause of revision surgery.[21,22]

REGULATION OF BODY WEIGHT: AN OVERVIEW

1. *Setpoint:* Large cohort studies examining the trajectory of body weight during adulthood show that most individuals with or without obesity maintain a body-weight between 0.3 and 0.5 kg/year.[23] However, this trajectory is significantly different among various racial and socioeconomic cohorts in society.[24] This relative constancy of body weight among all groups of individuals reinforces the role of the "setpoint" in maintaining weight and its vulnerability to change in response to interactions among homeostatic, genetic, and environmental factors. The setpoint, and therefore body weight, is vigorously defended by activating several counter-regulatory responses that aim to restore the energy balance to its baseline. These responses overlap, often reinforce one another, and differ in magnitude from one individual to the next. To understand the body's response to changes in energy balance, it is essential to outline the physiology of body-weight regulation.
2. Regulation of energy intake:
   a. *Role of the mediobasal hypothalamus:* The hypothalamus is regarded as the master sensor of energy balance. Two neighboring sets of neurons in the area of the arcuate nucleus in the mediobasal hypothalamus have been well investigated for their roles in energy intake and expenditure. Neurons that coexpress neuropeptide Y (NPY), Agouti-related peptide (AgRP), and γ-aminobutyric acid (GABA) are activated when energy balance is low, which stimulates feeding behavior.[25,26] The other group of neurons express pro-opiomelanocortin (POMC) and cocaine- and amphetamine-regulated transcript (CART), secrete the anorexigenic hormone α-melanocyte-stimulating hormone (αMSH). When energy stores are superfluous, peripheral signals such as leptin[27] stimulate POMC neurons causing them to release αMSH, which then activates melanocortin-4 receptors present on downstream (second-order neurons) in the paraventricular hypothalamic region, resulting in appetite suppression[28,29] (**Fig. 1**).

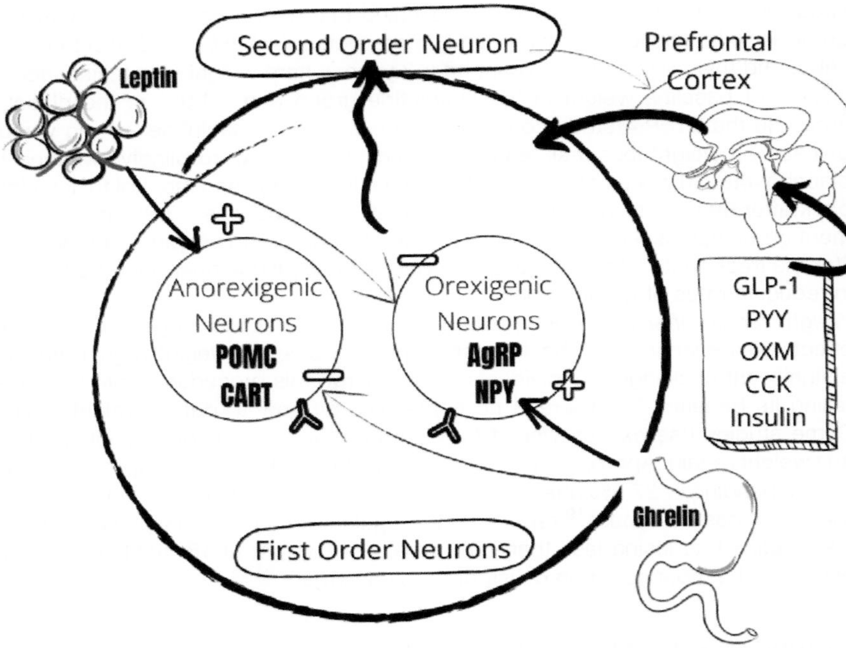

Fig. 1. Peripheral signals exert influence in the appetite centers of the mediobasal hypothalamus. Leptin secreted from adipocytes, stimulates anorexigenic neurons in the arcuate neurons, namely pro-opiomelanocortin and cocaine- and amphetamine-regulated transcript while inhibiting the orexigenic neurons Agouti-related peptide and neuropeptide Y. The net result is appetite suppression. Other peripheral hormones such as Ghrelin exert the opposite effects. These first-order neurons secrete neurotransmitters that act on second-order neurons which communicate with neuronal circuits in the prefrontal cortex that modify eating behavior. Furthermore, gut-related signals such as glucagon-like peptide-1, peptide tyrosine Y Y, oxyntomodulin, and insulin modulate appetite via afferent vagal signals acting in areas in the hindbrain such as the nucleus of the solitary tract.

b. *Role of the hindbrain and parabrachial nucleus:* The hindbrain receives afferent signals from various gut hormones conveyed through the vagus nerve that stimulate areas in the hindbrain, such as the nucleus of the solitary tract. From there, some neurons then project to the parabrachial nucleus, which contains calcium gene-related-peptide ($CGRP^{PBN}$) expressing neurons that are implicated in both satiety and satiation.[30] Bidirectional communication exists between the AgRP neurons in the hypothalamus and CGR^{PBN}, where activation of AgRP leads to inhibition of $CGRP^{PBN}$.[31] Stimulation of these CGR^{PBN} neurons has also been implicated in food aversion and the development of defensive responses and threat memory in animals.[32]
c. *Role of hormones and peripheral nutrient-sensing signals:* Leptin's role in regulating body fat was described in a landmark study published in 1994[33,34] and has since been a significant gateway to our current understanding of energy homeostasis. Levels of this adipokine hormone are proportionate to the fat mass and fluctuate in proportion to body weight in most individuals. Leptin acts as a satiety signal in the hypothalamus and activates the aforementioned neurons to suppress appetite. Although rare genetic causes of obesity associated with

hypoleptinemia may be treated by replacing leptin,[35] this has not been effective in treating the majority of people living with obesity. This implies a state of leptin-resistance, where despite a state of leptinemia, appetite and hunger signals remain elevated.[36] The gut-brain axis also plays a central role in body weight regulation and is the main drive for satiation.[37] A growing list of gut hormones has been implicated in appetite regulation. These hormones can be categorized broadly into orexigenic and anorexigenic. Orexigenic hormones include ghrelin[38,39] secreted by the gastric antrum and fundus, and motilin secreted by the small intestine.[40] Gut hormones well known to suppress appetite are glucagon-like peptide 1 (GLP-1) secreted by L-cells in the small intestine,[41,42] which is co-secreted with peptide tyrosine YY[43] and oxyntomodulin.[44,45] There is evidence that adipocytes in people with obesity may preferentially partition energy storage at the expense of lean mass in response to hormones, insulin, genetics, and the environment.[46,47]

d. *Role of environmental and behavioral influences on body weight:* The obesogenic environment has been implicated in the rise of obesity prevalence in youth and adults in many communities.[48,49] Hypothalamic inflammation resulting in injury has been linked to obesity and insulin resistance[50] in both humans and animals in response to high-fat, high-carbohydrate diets[51,52] presumably by altering the set point. In addition, food intake (stimulus) generates behavioral conditioning by activating potent neuronal circuits such as the dopamine, serotonin, cannabinoid, and opioid system. This translates into hedonic eating behaviors that override satiety signals generated by the hypothalamus. Furthermore, societal norms, stress, or habit result in inattentive eating behaviors in susceptible individuals, contributing to excess energy intake and the development of obesity.[53,54]

3. *Regulation of energy expenditure*: Bodyweight is determined by a balance between energy intake and energy expenditure in its basic form. In individuals with low baseline levels of PA, 60% of the energy expenditure is consumed by cardiorespiratory activity and maintenance of cellular gradients, 5% by the thermic effect of food and energy partitioning, and the remainder by low levels of planned and unplanned PA ("non-resting energy expenditure [NREE]"). Generally, the body's responses to changes in energy expenditure follow trends in energy intake. For example, overfeeding studies have found an increase in basal metabolic rate in response to expanding the fat and fat-free body mass.[55,56] Conversely, energy expenditure will drop when faced with energy restriction. However, adaptive thermogenesis causes the resting metabolic rate to decrease disproportionately to the caloric restriction,[57,58] which contributes to weight regain in the long term. A persistent mismatch between energy consumption and expenditure of only 3% will lead to an increase in body weight over time and result in obesity.[59]

PHYSIOLOGY OF THE WEIGHT-REDUCED STATE OF ITS IMPACT ON WEIGHT REGAIN

The fundamental principle of weight loss lies in achieving a negative energy balance, mainly through reducing caloric intake. In addition, active weight loss through negative energy balance and maintenance of a weight-reduced state through preserving energy equilibrium is associated with physiologic adaptations favoring hypometabolism and hyperphagia geared to defending the body's set point.[60] These can be broadly categorized into neuroendocrine systems, behavior, energy expenditure, and adipose tissue adaptations.

1. *Neuro-endocrine adaptations*: Changes in neurohormonal systems following weight loss in general favor increased appetite signals, decreased satiety,

enhanced food reward cues, and augmented energy storage. Compensatory increases in food consumption because of these changes contribute to weight regain. Validated mathematical models used to quantify the relative contribution of increased appetite versus decreased energy expenditure on food intake after weight loss have shown that appetite levels increased above baseline, leading to food consumption of ~100 kcal/d per kilogram of lost weight, whereas energy expenditure only reduced by 25 kcal/d per kg of lost weight.[61] This suggests that increased appetite likely plays a more significant role in weight regain than reduced energy expenditure. Adipokines, nutrient signaling hormones such as insulin and incretin hormone levels fluctuate in response to changes in body weight and may contribute to weight regain as well. However, studies have shown conflicting results. In a study by Sumithran and colleagues,[62] hunger-promoting hormones were measured during the weight-loss phase (8-week following a very low-calorie diet) and weight maintenance phase (week 10–52 of the study) in 50 participants with obesity. In addition to reporting hunger levels higher than baseline, levels of hormones that signal satiety (leptin, peptide YY, cholecystokinin, and insulin) remained lower than baseline. In contrast, the hunger hormones ghrelin, and gastric inhibitory peptide, which promotes energy storage, were higher. Changes in GLP-1 levels in response to different weight loss methods vary. After Roux-en-Y-gastric-bypass (RYGB), GLP-1 levels rise.[63,64] However, they remain unchanged and do not appear to mediate weight loss after sleeve gastrectomy or adjustable gastric banding in rodents.[65–67] The link between ghrelin levels and weight regain is also conflicting. In the DiRECT trial, ghrelin was measured in a sample of 253 participants who enrolled in a diet-mediated weight loss program. Higher ghrelin levels at 12 months predicted weight regain at 24 months after the intervention (for every 1.0 ng/mL increase, weight increased by 1.1%).[68] However, lower baseline ghrelin levels were associated with weight gain in other studies.[69,70] Leptin levels decline markedly during the active weight loss phase and proportionately to the new fat mass in the weight-reduced weight-maintenance phase.[34,71] Administration of exogenous leptin in physiologic doses to individuals who are in the weight-reduced, weight-maintenance state reverses many of the behavioral and energy changes that occur[71,72] (**Fig. 2**).

2. *Adaptations in energy expenditure*: Hypometabolism is a form of metabolic adaptation that occurs in response to weight loss and is characterized by a reduction in resting (REE) and NREE. The reduction in REE has been shown to persist as long as 1 year after weight loss is attained.[73] In fact, Hall and colleagues reported a significant ~600 kcal/d metabolic adaptation 6-year after weight loss in contestants from the program *The Biggest Loser*.[74,75] REE decreases after initial weight loss and during the weight maintenance phase after a 10% reduction in body weight [55,76]; however, it does not continue to decline after a weight loss from 10% to 20%. This is unlike NREE, which is also disproportionately reduced during and after a 10% loss of body weight but continues to decrease even further after a 20% weight loss. Adaptive thermogenesis refers to the decline in energy expenditure by the fat-free mass (skeletal muscle and organs), which occurs during weight loss.[77] The biological purpose of adaptive thermogenesis is to conserve energy and is mediated by changes in the sympathetic nervous system and declines in leptin and triiodothyronine levels (T3).[78] Animal studies have shown that after a period of caloric restriction, levels of deiodinase type 3 increase locally in the skeletal muscle, thereby reducing bioavailable T3 levels. Furthermore, deiodinase type 2 enzyme levels responsible for the activation of T3 are reduced, and a slower conversion of T3 from its precursor T4 also occurs. Last, there is a greater

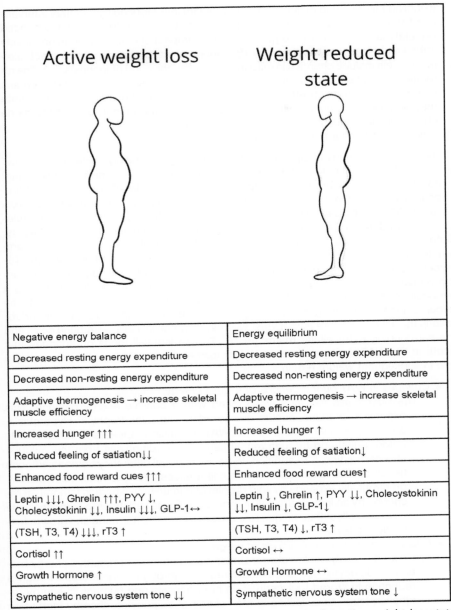

Active weight loss	Weight reduced state
Negative energy balance	Energy equilibrium
Decreased resting energy expenditure	Decreased resting energy expenditure
Decreased non-resting energy expenditure	Decreased non-resting energy expenditure
Adaptive thermogenesis → increase skeletal muscle efficiency	Adaptive thermogenesis → increase skeletal muscle efficiency
Increased hunger ↑↑↑	Increased hunger ↑
Reduced feeling of satiation↓↓	Reduced feeling of satiation↓
Enhanced food reward cues ↑↑↑	Enhanced food reward cues↑
Leptin ↓↓↓, Ghrelin ↑↑↑, PYY ↓, Cholecystokinin ↓↓, Insulin ↓↓↓, GLP-1↔	Leptin ↓ , Ghrelin ↑, PYY ↓↓, Cholecystokinin ↓↓, Insulin ↓, GLP-1↓
(TSH, T3, T4) ↓↓↓, rT3 ↑	(TSH, T3, T4) ↓, rT3 ↑
Cortisol ↑↑	Cortisol ↔
Growth Hormone ↑	Growth Hormone ↔
Sympathetic nervous system tone ↓↓	Sympathetic nervous system tone ↓

Fig. 2. Comparison between metabolic changes that occur in the active weight loss state and during the weight-reduced state. (*Data from* Refs.[62,73,76])

accumulation of the more-efficient isoforms of muscle fibers, namely MHC I isoform,[79] largely mediated by the decline leptin, and replacement of leptin seemed to ameliorate these changes and restore skeletal muscle function to baseline.[72] Furthermore, a study by Rosenbaum and colleagues[80] shown that repletion of T3 to individuals who had maintained a 10% weight loss induced by a dietary intervention for a duration of 5 weeks, reversed the metabolic profile favoring enhanced skeletal muscle efficiency, suggesting that the impact of declining leptin on muscle after weight loss was mediated by T3. Other molecular changes that impact skeletal muscle include changes in mitochondrial efficiency and biogenesis.[81,82] The alterations in skeletal muscle are geared to spare energy use and increase mechanical contraction efficiency so that a person in the weight-reduced state may acquire more contractile energy per calorie than an individual of the same characteristics who has not lost weight (see **Fig. 2**).

3. Adipose tissue adaptations (**Fig. 3**):

The primary function of adipocytes is to store energy in a highly efficient form; however, the biological function of this dynamic tissue expands beyond the evolutionary need for survival.[83] Anatomically, adipose tissue can be classified into visceral and subcutaneous. Additional classifications based on appearance include white adipose tissue (WAT) and beige/brown adipose tissue (BAT). Both classifications have relevance when determining their physiologic function and potential therapeutic targets. Both visceral and subcutaneous WAT have distinct developmental origins[84,85] and functions, and the overall WAT mass is central to determining overall body weight. Triglycerides, the main form of stored energy, are contained within the adipocyte and are the primary variable during periods of weight fluctuation.[86] In people exposed to a hypocaloric state, 75% of weight loss is attributed to loss of body fat.[55] Under these circumstances of weight gain and loss, WAT is required to undergo significant adaptations that involve mature adipocytes, vascular endothelial cells,[87] immune cells, and the surrounding extracellular matrix (ECM). This review will focus on changes that occur in the WAT during periods of weight loss and describe how they may play a role in subsequent weight regain.

- *Changes in WAT during periods of excess energy.*
  The WAT mass expands when faced with a positive energy balance. This expansion primarily occurs due to adipocyte hypertrophy.[88] Hyperplasia, another potential mechanism of WAT expansion, appears to occur mainly before adulthood through recruitment of pre-adipocytes from the vascular stromal fraction.[89] In addition, there are regional differences among adipose tissue depots when faced with nutrient excess; for example, visceral WAT preferentially expands by lipid droplet accumulation, whereas femoral fat responds by an increase in cell number size. These variations in adipose tissue changes reflect their unique responses to complex hormone and growth factor fluctuations.[87]
- *Changes in WAT during periods of weight loss.*
  a. *Changes to adipocyte volume:* Under circumstances of negative energy balance, adipocyte size is markedly reduced through volume loss through a reduction in stored triglycerides. In both animals and humans,[90] energy restriction leads to a decline in the volume of adipocytes, thereby increasing the percentage of small adipocytes and decreasing the number of large ones. Furthermore, when energy restriction is lifted, there will be a gradual restoration of adipocytes to their previous volumes, with little to no change in the overall number.
  b. *Changes in the number of adipocytes:* The overall population of adipocytes remains relatively stable throughout adulthood, where only 8% to 10% are replaced every year. The process of regenerating new adipocytes involves recruitment and proliferation of pre-adipocytes followed by their

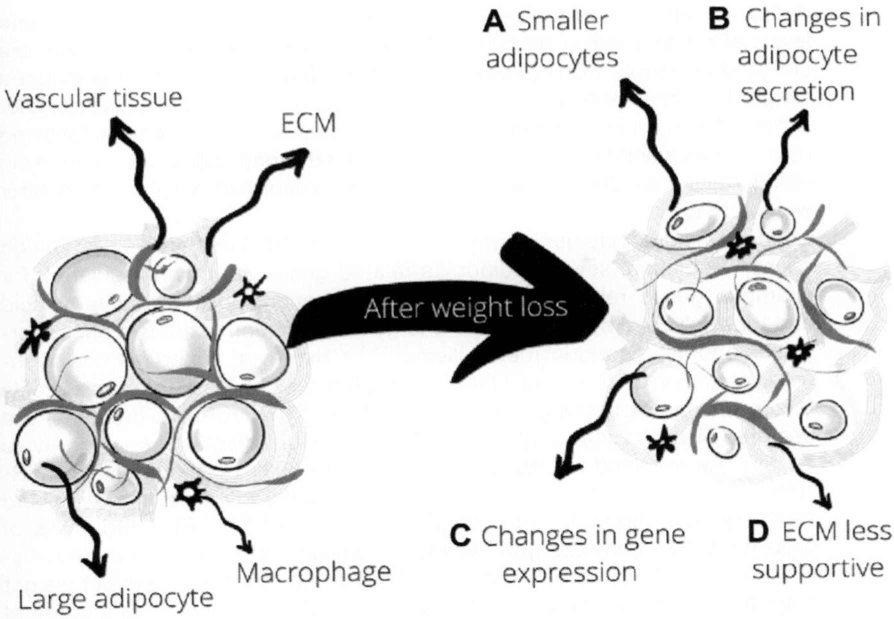

Fig. 3. Adipocyte changes after weight loss. Energy restriction elicits a series of changes in in adipose tissue. (A) Adipocytes lose stored triglycerides and thereby volume, becoming smaller in size.[90] Weight regain occurs mainly by refilling mature adipocytes rather than recruitment of new pre-adipocytes from the vasculature. (B) Adipokine secretion such as leptin and retinol binding protein (RBP) change after weight loss. Studies have found a correlation between RBP levels and weight regain.[105] (C) Reduction in adipocyte volume also induces a series of changes in gene expression, such as those related to adipocyte proliferation, energy consumption,[106] and energy partitioning.7,108 MicroRNAs are also secreted by adipocytes, some which correlate with weight regain.[115] (D) The extracellular matrix becomes unable to support smaller adipocytes after weight loss, and must undergo considerable remodeling which creates activation of stress signals that favor energy partitioning to the adipocyte.[116]

differentiation into mature cells capable of storing lipid droplets. However, the process of clearing mature adipocytes is not well defined but seems to involve macrophages[91,92] driven by complex regulatory signals, including hormones and growth factors.[93] It is not yet clear whether the weight-reduced state favors a shift in adipose tissue turnover to a state of new adipocyte formation over clearance; therefore, it seems that weight regain is primarily a function of refilling mature adipocytes rather than forming new ones.

c. *Changes in adipokine secretion:* Obesity is characterized by leptin resistance and hyperleptinemia.[94] Leptin secretion decreases during periods of weight loss[93]; however, evidence suggests that the magnitude of leptin decline is disproportionate to what would be anticipated from the reduction in WAT mass.[93,95,96] Leptin influences homeostatic centers in the hypothalamus. Decline in leptin levels enhances the secretion of NPY, corticotropin-releasing peptide,[97–99] and Agouti-related peptide (AgRP)[100–102] to promote a positive energy balance. Moreover, reduced leptin levels decrease the expression of POMC, which favors a negative energy balance.[102] The combined effect of these neurohormonal changes is weight gain. Plasma levels of retinol-binding protein 4 (RBP4), a pro-inflammatory adipokine, are elevated in people with obesity and decline after surgical and diet-induced weight-loss interventions.[103,104] In a randomized control trial involving either a low-calorie diet for 12 weeks or a very low-calorie diet for 5 weeks, followed by a 4-week weight maintenance phase and a 9-month follow-up, changes in RBP4 measured during these study phases predicted weight regain after weight loss.[105]

d. *Changes in adipocyte gene expression and micro RNA (miRNA) levels:* During energy restriction, several adipocyte-related genes are down-regulated, for example, genes related to adipocyte proliferation (unsaturated fatty acid and triacylglycerol synthesis), and energy consumption (oxidative phosphorylation and mitochondrial metabolism).[106,107] However, during periods of energy restriction and weight stabilization after weight loss, the gene profile favors energy partitioning and storage of fat.[108] MicroRNAs (miRNAs) are secreted by adipocytes and have local and systemic effects. Circulating levels of miRNAs secreted by adipocytes constitute 80% of all circulating miRNAs.[109] Their effects include adipose tissue differentiation, browning and thermogenesis, lipolysis, and overall homeostasis.[110–112] Elevated levels of certain miRNAs correlate with obesity-related diseases such as insulin resistance and metabolic liver disease,[113,114] whereas others may predict weight responses to weight loss interventions or metabolic health.[109] In a study of 78 subjects with obesity who underwent two different diet-induced weight-loss interventions, circulating levels of 86 miRNAs were measured and compared with normal-weight controls. Seven miRNAs were found to predict participants' responses to the weight-loss intervention.[115] Although there is ample evidence of the various biological influences of miRNA on adipocyte function, further studies are needed to elucidate the impact of miRNAs on weight regain.

e. *Changes to adipose tissue ECM:* During weight loss, the ECM supporting adipocytes undergo considerable remodeling to accommodate smaller adipocytes.[116] Development and maintenance of the ECM is an energy-consuming process, therefore under circumstances of energy restriction, the adipocytes' ability to maintain the ECM is impaired, creating stress signals[117] such as inhibition of lipolysis,[118] upregulation of focal adhesion pathways,[119] increased levels of heat shock proteins (HSP) 60 and HSP70,[120] and sex-specific changes in stress-related gene expression.[121] These changes seem to promote nutrient partitioning and fat re-accumulation in the adipocytes.

STRATEGIES TO ANTICIPATE AND MITIGATE WEIGHT REGAIN

1. Behavioral predictors of weight regain:

An important aspect of weight regain lies in behavioral factors that are central to food-seeking and intake. Certain personality traits have been shown to correlate with eating patterns and health outcomes. The Five-Factor Model (FFM) of personality is a well-studied questionnaire that measures neuroticism, extroversion, openness to experience, agreeableness, and conscientiousness, which has been linked to the risk of developing obesity.[122,123] Individuals who scored higher on the neuroticism scale tended to have body weights in the abnormal range (under or overweight),[124] and those who scored lower on the conscientiousness scale had an increase in BMI over 14 years of middle-adulthood years.[122] Sutin and colleagues[125] assessed personality traits from the FFM in a cohort of 1988 individuals enrolled in a longitudinal study that spanned 50 years and measured the BMI trajectory. They found the strongest correlation with BMI was with impulsivity facets where those who scored in the top 10% of the scale weighed 11 kg more than those who scored at the bottom 10%. Using personality assessment questionnaires may aid in predicting those who may be prone to weight regain so that interventions targeting behavioral changes can be an early part of weight loss intervention. Other behavioral domains that may be linked to weight regain are "passive" (mindless) eating, where trifle amounts of food consumption occur regularly, creating small daily positive gains in energy, or "active" eating driven by cravings, hedonic, or emotional eating. Multiple studies using functional MRI have shown changes in the reward centers of the brain in individuals who have obesity[126] both before and after weight loss.[127] Using imaging to detect patterns of heightened signals in reward centers may predict who may be at risk for weight regain so that interventions with behavioral and pharmacotherapy interventions can be initiated early on.

2. Predictors of weight gain after metabolic surgery:

   A useful algorithm developed by Istfan and colleagues[128] provides clinicians with a clinical management tool to aid in early recognition and intervention of weight regain in patients who have had bariatric surgery (**Fig. 4**). They aimed to identify those at greatest risk for regaining greater than 5% of their nadir weight in 6 months, or greater than 10% of nadir weight in less than a year, to provide effective and early intervention. Based on this assessment, weight regain was defined as any weight that had increased above nadir weight. The authors classified weight regain as mild (0.2%–<0.5%), moderate (0.5%–1.0%), and severe (>1.0%) in a 30-day period. Those in the moderate and severe groups should be considered for pharmacotherapy and evaluation of the upper gastrointestinal anatomy using techniques such as a barium swallow or upper GI endoscopy, to rule out fistulas and assess the size of the remnant stomach. . All patients should receive ongoing medical nutrition therapy, PA, and behavioral counseling.

3. Genotype predictors of the magnitude and rate of weight loss and weight regain:

   Genome-wide associations have identified over 1000 single-nucleotide polymorphisms (SNPs) associated with markers of adiposity such as BMI, birth weight, waist to hip ratio, and extreme obesity.[129,130] Genetic variants in participants enrolled in the DPP[131] and Look AHEAD[132] were analyzed to determine the association between genetic loci and weight loss at 1 year and weight regain at 2 to 4 years in those who lost at least 3% or more of their total body weight.[133,134] Some SNPs correlated with initial weight loss, such as mitochondrial proliferator-activated receptor 3 (*MTIF3*), neural growth regulator 1 (*NEGR1*), peroxisome proliferator-activated receptor γ and Transcription initiation factor IIE subunit β (*TFA2β*) but not weight regain. Other SNPs such as brain-derived neurotrophic factor (*BDNF*) and fat mass and obesity-associated gene (*FTO*)[134,135] were linked to weight regain. Although these genotype associations may serve as therapeutic targets or predictors of outcomes, more studies are needed to elucidate their function and identify how these genetic variants interact with the environment and social-emotional context in which these genes exist, that is, the "norm of reaction".[136]

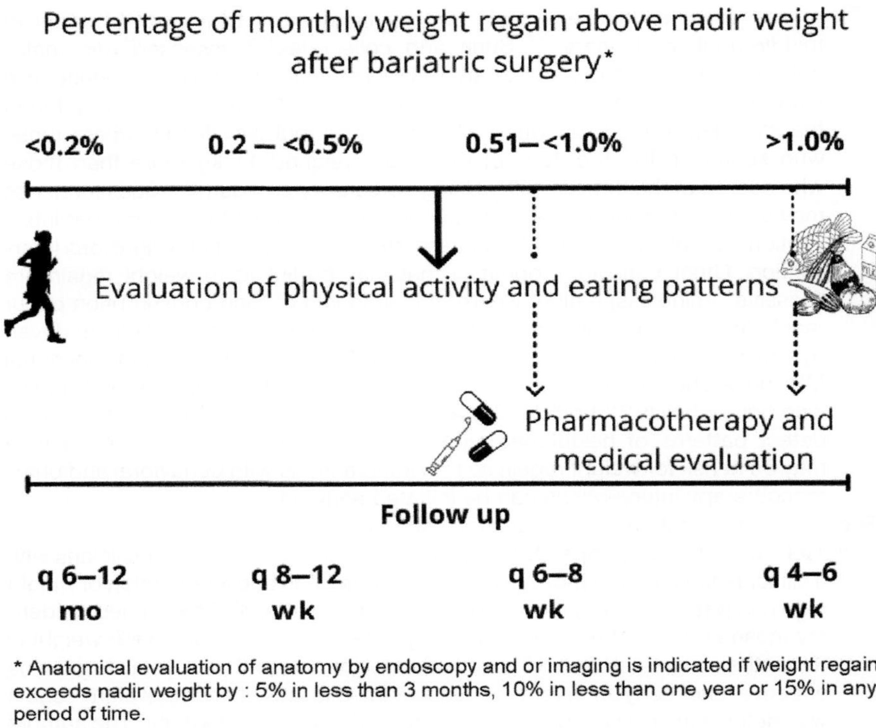

Fig. 4. Percentage of monthly weight regain above nadir weight after bariatric surgery* (*Adapted from* Istfan NW, Lipartia M, Anderson WA, Hess DT, Apovian CM. Approach to the Patient: Management of the Post-Bariatric Surgery Patient With Weight Regain. J Clin Endocrinol Metab. 2021;106(1):251-263; with permission.)

Patient-Related Outcomes and Weight Regain

Weight loss has been associated with improvements in outcomes related to health-related quality of life (HRQoL),[137] type 2 diabetes, sleep apnea, diabetes, and dyslipidemia.[138,139] Several studies have shown that living with obesity is associated with adverse quality of life measures.[140,141] However, the impact of weight regain on patient-related outcomes has not been researched as thoroughly. In one study investigating the effect of weight regain on HRQoL involving 40,098 women from the Nurses' Health Study, those who gained between 5 and 20 lb over 4 years had decreased physical function and vitality and increased body weight irrespective of their baseline weight.[142] Another study comparing the impact of weight regain and weight loss on HRQoL measures in 122 subjects enrolled in a weight management program who received phentermine-fenfluramine and lost $\geq$5% of their baseline weight showed that those who subsequently regained $\geq$ 5% of their weight had impaired measures of HRQoL.[143] Weight cycling, where individuals undergo periods of weight loss followed by weight gain, has been a focus of studies attempting to elucidate whether or not its effects are deleterious to health above and beyond the long-term impact of obesity. Animal studies have shown a negative impact of repeatedly losing and regaining weight on bone health[144] and glucose metabolism.[145] In human studies, most studies have focused on mortality as an outcome of weight cycling however no significant association has been found between periodic weight regain after weight loss and mortality regardless of the person's BMI.[146] However, inconsistencies exist in the literature related to the association between weight cycling and cardiovascular biomarkers, glucose metabolism, inflammatory markers, cancer, and body composition. Many variables potentially confound these results, including weight loss methods, sample size, duration of weight loss before weight gain, number of weight loss–regain cycles, gender, age, and race. Finally, weight regain after bariatric surgery offers a unique opportunity to study the impact of weight regain on patient outcomes because of the weight-independent benefits conferred by the metabolic changes that ensue after metabolic surgery. In a prospective cohort study of 1406 adults who had RYGB, weight regain measured as a percentage of maximum weight gained after reaching a nadir had the strongest association with progression of diabetes, hypertension, and the decline in physical HRQoL.[147] In conclusion, weight regain after weight loss has negative consequences on several facets pertaining to HRQoL metrics, such as physical function, mental health, self-esteem, sexual life, public distress, work overall well-being. It is unknown whether the individuals' age, race, gender, number of weight cycles, mode of weight loss, or other factors play a role in the outcomes of weight regain.

CLINICS CARE POINTS

- It is important to recognize that obesity is a chronic disease, offer patients evidence-based treatment, and avoid blaming individuals for inadequate responses to weight-management interventions.
- When recommending weight management interventions, patients should be monitored regularly for an adequate response to treatment, and offered alternatives or supplemental treatment when appropriate.
- After patients attain weight loss, long-term follow-up is needed because of the risk for recidivism driven by the physiologic drive to regain the weight.
- Acknowledging variations in personality traits, genetics, physiology, and environmental circumstances is an essential component of any weight management program to maximize therapeutic impact and minimize obesity-related biases that people living with obesity often face.

DISCLOSURE

S. Hafida: no disclosure. C. Apovian: Has participated on advisory boards for Altimmune, Inc., Cowen and Company, LLC, Gelesis, Srl., L-Nutra, Inc., NeuroBo Pharmaceuticals, Inc., Novo Nordisk, Inc., Pain Script Corporation, Riverview School, Rhythm Pharmaceuticals, and Xeno Biosciences. Dr C. Apovian has received research funding from the NIH, PCORI and GI Dynamics, Inc.

REFERENCES

1. Grover A, Joshi A. An overview of chronic disease models: a systematic literature review. Glob J Health Sci 2014;7(2):210–27.
2. Obesity and overweight. Available at: https://www.who.int/news-room/fact-sheets/detail/obesity-and-overweight. Accessed November 3, 2021.
3. Santos I, Sniehotta FF, Marques MM, et al. Prevalence of personal weight control attempts in adults: a systematic review and meta-analysis. Obes Rev 2017; 18(1):32–50.

4. National Weight Control Registry. Available at: http://www.nwcr.ws/. Accessed February 25, 2022.
5. Thomas JG, Bond DS, Phelan S, et al. Weight-loss maintenance for 10 years in the National Weight Control Registry. Am J Prev Med 2014;46(1):17–23.
6. Catenacci VA, Odgen L, Phelan S, et al. Dietary habits and weight maintenance success in high versus low exercisers in the National Weight Control Registry. J Phys Act Health 2014;11(8):1540–8.
7. Apovian CM, Aronne LJ, Bessesen DH, et al. Pharmacological management of obesity: an endocrine Society clinical practice guideline. J Clin Endocrinol Metab 2015;100(2):342–62.
8. Goodpaster BH, Delany JP, Otto AD, et al. Effects of diet and physical activity interventions on weight loss and cardiometabolic risk factors in severely obese adults: a randomized trial. JAMA 2010;304(16):1795–802.
9. Look AHEAD Research Group, Wing RR. Long-term effects of a lifestyle intervention on weight and cardiovascular risk factors in individuals with type 2 diabetes mellitus: four-year results of the Look AHEAD trial. Arch Intern Med 2010; 170(17):1566–75.
10. Diabetes Prevention Program (DPP) Research Group. The Diabetes Prevention Program (DPP): description of lifestyle intervention. Diabetes Care 2002;25(12): 2165–71.
11. Look AHEAD Research Group. Eight-year weight losses with an intensive lifestyle intervention: the look AHEAD study. Obesity 2014;22(1):5–13.
12. Christiansen T, Bruun JM, Madsen EL, et al. Weight loss maintenance in severely obese adults after an intensive lifestyle intervention: 2- to 4-year follow-up. Obesity 2007;15(2):413–20.
13. le Roux CW, Astrup A, Fujioka K, et al. 3 years of liraglutide versus placebo for type 2 diabetes risk reduction and weight management in individuals with prediabetes: a randomised, double-blind trial. Lancet 2017;389(10077):1399–409
14. Rubino D, Abrahamsson N, Davies M, et al. Effect of Continued Weekly Subcutaneous Semaglutide vs Placebo on Weight Loss Maintenance in Adults With Overweight or Obesity: The STEP 4 Randomized Clinical Trial. JAMA 2021 325(14):1414–25.
15. El Ansari W, Elhag W. Weight Regain and Insufficient Weight Loss After Bariatric Surgery: Definitions, Prevalence, Mechanisms, Predictors, Prevention and Management Strategies, and Knowledge Gaps-a Scoping Review. Obes Surg 2021 31(4):1755–66.
16. Adams TD, Davidson LE, Litwin SE, et al. Weight and Metabolic Outcomes 12 Years after Gastric Bypass. N Engl J Med 2017;377(12):1143–55.
17. Sjöström L, Lindroos AK, Peltonen M, et al. Lifestyle, diabetes, and cardiovascular risk factors 10 years after bariatric surgery. N Engl J Med 2004;351(26) 2683–93.
18. Clapp B, Wynn M, Martyn C, et al. Long term (7 or more years) outcomes of the sleeve gastrectomy: a meta-analysis. Surg Obes Relat Dis 2018;14(6):741–7.
19. Courcoulas AP, King WC, Belle SH, et al. Seven-Year Weight Trajectories and Health Outcomes in the Longitudinal Assessment of Bariatric Surgery (LABS Study. JAMA Surg 2018;153(5):427–34.
20. Nedelcu M, Khwaja HA, Rogula TG. Weight regain after bariatric surgery—how should it be defined? Surg Obes Relat Dis 2016;12(5):1129–30.
21. Andalib A, Alamri H, Almuhanna Y, et al. Short-term outcomes of revisional surgery after sleeve gastrectomy: a comparative analysis of re-sleeve, Roux en-Y

gastric bypass, duodenal switch (Roux en-Y and single-anastomosis). Surg Endosc 2021;35(8):4644–52.
22. Hernández LA, Guilbert L, Sepúlveda EM, et al. Causes of revisional surgery, reoperations, and readmissions after bariatric surgery. Rev Gastroenterol Mex 2021. https://doi.org/10.1016/j.rgmxen.2021.12.006.
23. Zheng Y, Manson JE, Yuan C, et al. Associations of Weight Gain From Early to Middle Adulthood With Major Health Outcomes Later in Life. JAMA 2017;318(3): 255–69.
24. Yang YC, Walsh CE, Johnson MP, et al. Life-course trajectories of body mass index from adolescence to old age: Racial and educational disparities. Proc Natl Acad Sci U S A 2021;118(17).
25. Aponte Y, Atasoy D, Sternson SM. AGRP neurons are sufficient to orchestrate feeding behavior rapidly and without training. Nat Neurosci 2011;14(3):351–5.
26. Kim JD, Leyva S, Diano S. Hormonal regulation of the hypothalamic melanocortin system. Front Physiol 2014;5:480. https://doi.org/10.3389/fphys.2014.00480.
27. Schwartz MW, Seeley RJ, Woods SC, et al. Leptin increases hypothalamic proopiomelanocortin mRNA expression in the rostral arcuate nucleus. Diabetes 1997;46(12):2119–23.
28. Sternson SM, Eiselt AK. Three Pillars for the Neural Control of Appetite. Annu Rev Physiol 2017;79:401–23.
29. Berthoud HR, Münzberg H, Morrison CD. Blaming the Brain for Obesity: Integration of Hedonic and Homeostatic Mechanisms. Gastroenterology 2017;152(7): 1728–38.
30. Grill HJ, Hayes MR. Hindbrain neurons as an essential hub in the neuroanatomically distributed control of energy balance. Cell Metab 2012;16(3):296–309.
31. Roman CW, Derkach VA, Palmiter RD. Genetically and functionally defined NTS to PBN brain circuits mediating anorexia. Nat Commun 2016;7:11905.
32. Han S, Soleiman MT, Soden ME, et al. Elucidating an Affective Pain Circuit that Creates a Threat Memory. Cell 2015;162(2):363–74.
33. Zhang Y, Proenca R, Maffei M, et al. Positional cloning of the mouse obese gene and its human homologue. Nature 1994;372(6505):425–32.
34. Leibel RL. The role of leptin in the control of body weight. Nutr Rev 2002;60(10 Pt 2). S15-S19; discussion S68-S84, 85-87.
35. Farooqi IS, O'Rahilly S. Monogenic human obesity syndromes. Recent Prog Horm Res 2004;59:409–24.
36. Myers MG Jr, Leibel RL, Seeley RJ, et al. Obesity and leptin resistance: distinguishing cause from effect. Trends Endocrinol Metab 2010;21(11):643–51.
37. Lean MEJ, Malkova D. Altered gut and adipose tissue hormones in overweight and obese individuals: cause or consequence? Int J Obes 2016;40(4):622–32.
38. Pradhan G, Samson SL, Sun Y. Ghrelin: much more than a hunger hormone. Curr Opin Clin Nutr Metab Care 2013;16(6):619–24.
39. Sato T, Nakamura Y, Shiimura Y, et al. Structure, regulation and function of ghrelin. J Biochem 2012;151(2):119–28. Available at: https://academic.oup.com/jb/article-abstract/151/2/119/2182660.
40. Deloose E, Verbeure W, Depoortere I, et al. Motilin: from gastric motility stimulation to hunger signalling. Nat Rev Endocrinol 2019;15(4):238–50.
41. Thorens B. Expression cloning of the pancreatic beta cell receptor for the glucoincretin hormone glucagon-like peptide 1. Proc Natl Acad Sci U S A 1992; 89(18):8641–5.
42. Drucker DJ. GLP-1 physiology informs the pharmacotherapy of obesity. Mol Metab 2022;57:101351.

43. Karra E, Chandarana K, Batterham RL. The role of peptide YY in appetite regulation and obesity. J Physiol 2009;587(1):19–25.
44. Dakin CL, Gunn I, Small CJ, et al. Oxyntomodulin inhibits food intake in the rat. Endocrinology 2001;142(10):4244–50.
45. Wynne K, Park AJ, Small CJ, et al. Subcutaneous oxyntomodulin reduces body weight in overweight and obese subjects: a double-blind, randomized, controlled trial. Diabetes 2005;54(8):2390–5.
46. Muoio DM, Dohm GL, Fiedorek FT Jr, et al. Leptin directly alters lipid partitioning in skeletal muscle. Diabetes 1997;46(8):1360–3.
47. Archer E, Pavela G, McDonald S, et al. Cell-Specific "Competition for Calories" Drives Asymmetric Nutrient-Energy Partitioning, Obesity, and Metabolic Diseases in Human and Non-human Animals. Front Physiol 2018;9:1053. https://doi.org/10.3389/fphys.2018.01053.
48. Wilding S, Ziauddeen N, Smith D, et al. Are environmental area characteristics at birth associated with overweight and obesity in school-aged children? Findings from the SLOPE (Studying Lifecourse Obesity PrEdictors) population-based cohort in the south of England. BMC Med 2020;18(1):43.
49. Inoue Y, Howard AG, Thompson AL, et al. Secular change in the association between urbanisation and abdominal adiposity in China (1993-2011). J Epidemiol Community Health 2018;72(6):484–90.
50. Jais A, Brüning JC. Hypothalamic inflammation in obesity and metabolic disease. J Clin Invest 2017;127(1):24–32.
51. Thaler JP, Yi CX, Schur EA, et al. Obesity is associated with hypothalamic injury in rodents and humans. J Clin Invest 2012;122(1):153–62.
52. Cazettes F, Cohen JI, Yau PL, et al. Obesity-mediated inflammation may damage the brain circuit that regulates food intake. Brain Res 2011;1373:101–9.
53. Atkinson TJ. Central and peripheral neuroendocrine peptides and signalling in appetite regulation: considerations for obesity pharmacotherapy. Obes Rev 2008;9(2):108–20.
54. Cota D, Tschöp MH, Horvath TL, et al. Cannabinoids, opioids and eating behavior: the molecular face of hedonism? Brain Res Rev 2006;51(1):85–107.
55. Leibel RL, Rosenbaum M, Hirsch J. Changes in energy expenditure resulting from altered body weight. N Engl J Med 1995;332(10):621–8.
56. Joosen AMCP, Westerterp KR. Energy expenditure during overfeeding. Nutr Metab 2006;3:25.
57. Camps SGJA, Verhoef SPM, Westerterp KR. Weight loss, weight maintenance, and adaptive thermogenesis. Am J Clin Nutr 2013;97(5):990–4.
58. Ravussin E, Ryan DH. Energy expenditure and weight control: Is the biggest loser the best loser? Obesity 2016;24(8):1607–8.
59. Schwartz MW, Seeley RJ, Zeltser LM, et al. Obesity Pathogenesis: An Endocrine Society Scientific Statement. Endocr Rev 2017;38(4):267–96.
60. Aronne LJ, Hall KD, Jakicic J, et al. Describing the weight-Reduced State: Physiology, behavior, and interventions. Obesity 2021;29(Suppl S1):S9–24.
61. Polidori D, Sanghvi A, Seeley RJ, et al. How Strongly Does Appetite Counter Weight Loss? Quantification of the Feedback Control of Human Energy Intake. Obes 2016;24(11):2289–95.
62. Sumithran P, Prendergast LA, Delbridge E, et al. Long-term persistence of hormonal adaptations to weight loss. N Engl J Med 2011;365(17):1597–604.
63. Kellum JM, Kuemmerle JF, O'Dorisio TM, et al. Gastrointestinal hormone responses to meals before and after gastric bypass and vertical banded gastroplasty. Ann Surg 1990;211(6):763–70.

64. le Roux CW, Welbourn R, Werling M, et al. Gut hormones as mediators of appetite and weight loss after Roux-en-Y gastric bypass. Ann Surg 2007;246(5):780–5.
65. Wilson-Pérez HE, Chambers AP, Ryan KK, et al. Vertical sleeve gastrectomy is effective in two genetic mouse models of glucagon-like Peptide 1 receptor deficiency. Diabetes 2013;62(7):2380–5.
66. Mul JD, Begg DP, Alsters SIM, et al. Effect of vertical sleeve gastrectomy in melanocortin receptor 4-deficient rats. Am J Physiol Endocrinol Metab 2012;303(1):E103–10.
67. Shah M, Vella A. Effects of GLP-1 on appetite and weight. Rev Endocr Metab Disord 2014;15(3):181–7.
68. Thom G, McIntosh A, Messow CM, et al. Weight loss-induced increase in fasting ghrelin concentration is a predictor of weight regain: Evidence from the Diabetes Remission Clinical Trial (DiRECT). Diabetes Obes Metab 2020. https://doi.org/10.1111/dom.14274.
69. Crujeiras AB, Goyenechea E, Abete I, et al. Weight regain after a diet-induced loss is predicted by higher baseline leptin and lower ghrelin plasma levels. J Clin Endocrinol Metab 2010;95(11):5037–44.
70. Garcia JM, Iyer D, Poston WSC, et al. Rise of plasma ghrelin with weight loss is not sustained during weight maintenance. Obesity 2006;14(10):1716–23.
71. Rosenbaum M, Sy M, Pavlovich K, et al. Leptin reverses weight loss–induced changes in regional neural activity responses to visual food stimuli. J Clin Invest 2008;118(7):2583–91.
72. Rosenbaum M, Goldsmith R, Bloomfield D, et al. Low-dose leptin reverses skeletal muscle, autonomic, and neuroendocrine adaptations to maintenance of reduced weight. J Clin Invest 2005;115(12):3579–86.
73. Rosenbaum M, Hirsch J, Gallagher DA, et al. Long-term persistence of adaptive thermogenesis in subjects who have maintained a reduced body weight. Am J Clin Nutr 2008;88(4):906–12.
74. Hall KD. Energy compensation and metabolic adaptation: "The Biggest Loser" study reinterpreted. Obes 2022;30(1):11–3.
75. Fothergill E, Guo J, Howard L, et al. Persistent metabolic adaptation 6 years after "The Biggest Loser" competition. Obes 2016;24(8):1612–9.
76. Rosenbaum M, Leibel RL. Models of energy homeostasis in response to maintenance of reduced body weight. Obesity 2016;24(8):1620–9.
77. Müller MJ, Bosy-Westphal A. Adaptive thermogenesis with weight loss in humans. Obesity 2013;21(2):218–28.
78. Müller MJ, Enderle J, Pourhassan M, et al. Metabolic adaptation to caloric restriction and subsequent refeeding: the Minnesota Starvation Experiment revisited. Am J Clin Nutr 2015;102(4):807–19.
79. De Andrade PBM, Neff LA, Strosova MK, et al. Caloric restriction induces energy-sparing alterations in skeletal muscle contraction, fiber composition and local thyroid hormone metabolism that persist during catch-up fat upon refeeding. Front Physiol 2015;6:254.
80. Rosenbaum M, Goldsmith RL, Haddad F, et al. Triiodothyronine and leptin repletion in humans similarly reverse weight-loss-induced changes in skeletal muscle. Am J Physiol Endocrinol Metab 2018;315(5):E771–9.
81. Civitarese AE, Carling S, Heilbronn LK, et al. Calorie restriction increases muscle mitochondrial biogenesis in healthy humans. Plos Med 2007;4(3):e76.

82. Sparks LM, Redman LM, Conley KE, et al. Effects of 12 Months of Caloric Restriction on Muscle Mitochondrial Function in Healthy Individuals. J Clin Endocrinol Metab 2017;102(1):111–21.
83. Cypess AM. Reassessing Human Adipose Tissue. N Engl J Med 2022;386(8): 768–79.
84. Chen L, Dai YM, Ji CB, et al. MiR-146b is a regulator of human visceral preadipocyte proliferation and differentiation and its expression is altered in humar obesity. Mol Cell Endocrinol 2014;393(1–2):65–74.
85. Long JZ, Svensson KJ, Tsai L, et al. A smooth muscle-like origin for beige adipocytes. Cell Metab 2014;19(5):810–20.
86. Lee MJ, Wu Y, Fried SK. Adipose tissue remodeling in pathophysiology of obesity. Curr Opin Clin Nutr Metab Care 2010;13(4):371–6.
87. Lee MJ, Wu Y, Fried SK. Adipose tissue heterogeneity: Implication of depot differences in adipose tissue for obesity complications. Mol Aspects Med 2013 34(1):1–11.
88. Spalding KL, Arner E, Westermark PO, et al. Dynamics of fat cell turnover in humans. Nature 2008;453(7196):783–7.
89. Tchkonia T, Thomou T, Zhu Y, et al. Mechanisms and metabolic implications o regional differences among fat depots. Cell Metab 2013;17(5):644–56.
90. Maclean PS, Bergouignan A, Cornier MA, et al. Biology's response to dieting the impetus for weight regain. Am J Physiol Regul Integr Comp Physiol 2011 301(3):R581–600.
91. Capel F, Klimcáková E, Viguerie N, et al. Macrophages and adipocytes in hu man obesity: adipose tissue gene expression and insulin sensitivity during cal orie restriction and weight stabilization. Diabetes 2009;58(7):1558–67.
92. Cinti S, Mitchell G, Barbatelli G, et al. Adipocyte death defines macrophag localization and function in adipose tissue of obese mice and humans. J Lipic Res 2005;46(11):2347–55.
93. Rosenbaum M, Nicolson M, Hirsch J, et al. Effects of weight change on plasm leptin concentrations and energy expenditure. J Clin Endocrinol Metab 1997 82(11):3647–54.
94. Mendoza-Herrera K, Florio AA, Moore M, et al. The Leptin System and Diet: Mini Review of the Current Evidence. Front Endocrinol 2021;12:749050.
95. Arner P, Spalding KL. Fat cell turnover in humans. Biochem Biophys Res Com mun 2010;396(1):101–4.
96. Strohacker K, McCaffery JM, MacLean PS, et al. Adaptations of leptin, ghrelin o insulin during weight loss as predictors of weight regain: a review of current liter ature. Int J Obes 2014;38(3):388–96.
97. Schwartz MW, Baskin DG, Bukowski TR, et al. Specificity of leptin action o elevated blood glucose levels and hypothalamic neuropeptide Y gene expres sion in ob/ob mice. Diabetes 1996;45(4):531–5.
98. Jang M, Mistry A, Swick AG, et al. Leptin rapidly inhibits hypothalamic neuro peptide Y secretion and stimulates corticotropin-releasing hormone secretio in adrenalectomized mice. J Nutr 2000;130(11):2813–20.
99. Wang Q, Bing C, Al-Barazanji K, et al. Interactions between leptin and hypotha lamic neuropeptide Y neurons in the control of food intake and energy homec stasis in the rat. Diabetes 1997;46(3):335–41.
100. Gonçalves GHM, Li W, Garcia AVCG, et al. Hypothalamic agouti-related peptid neurons and the central melanocortin system are crucial mediators of leptin antidiabetic actions. Cell Rep 2014;7(4):1093–103.

101. Sheffer-Babila S, Sun Y, Israel DD, et al. Agouti-related peptide plays a critical role in leptin's effects on female puberty and reproduction. Am J Physiol Endocrinol Metab 2013;305(12):E1512–20.
102. Page-Wilson G, Meece K, White A, et al. Proopiomelanocortin, agouti-related protein, and leptin in human cerebrospinal fluid: correlations with body weight and adiposity. Am J Physiol Endocrinol Metab 2015;309(5):E458–65.
103. Haider DG, Schindler K, Prager G, et al. Serum retinol-binding protein 4 is reduced after weight loss in morbidly obese subjects. J Clin Endocrinol Metab 2007;92(3):1168–71.
104. Janke J, Engeli S, Boschmann M, et al. Retinol-binding protein 4 in human obesity. Diabetes 2006;55(10):2805–10.
105. Vink RG, Roumans NJ, Mariman EC, et al. Dietary weight loss-induced changes in RBP4, FFA, and ACE predict weight regain in people with overweight and obesity. Phys Rep 2017;5(21). https://doi.org/10.14814/phy2.13450.
106. Viguerie N, Vidal H, Arner P, et al. Adipose tissue gene expression in obese subjects during low-fat and high-fat hypocaloric diets. Diabetologia 2005;48(1): 123–31.
107. Adipose tissue transcriptome reflects variations between subjects with continued weight loss and subjects regaining weight 6 mo after caloric restriction independent of energy intake. Am J Clin Nutr 2010;92(4):975–84. Available at: https://academic.oup.com/ajcn/article-abstract/92/4/975/4597621.
108. MacLean PS, Higgins JA, Giles ED, et al. The role for adipose tissue in weight regain after weight loss. Obes Rev 2015;16(Suppl 1):45–54.
109. Kurylowicz A. microRNAs in Human Adipose Tissue Physiology and Dysfunction. Cells 2021;10(12). https://doi.org/10.3390/cells10123342.
110. Gharanei S, Shabir K, Brown JE, et al. Regulatory microRNAs in Brown, Brite and White Adipose Tissue. Cells 2020;9(11):2489.
111. Ortega FJ, Moreno-Navarrete JM, Pardo G, et al. MiRNA expression profile of human subcutaneous adipose and during adipocyte differentiation. PLoS One 2010;5(2):e9022.
112. Thomou T, Mori MA, Dreyfuss JM, et al. Adipose-derived circulating miRNAs regulate gene expression in other tissues. Nature 2017;542(7642):450–5.
113. Estep M, Armistead D, Hossain N, et al. Differential expression of miRNAs in the visceral adipose tissue of patients with non-alcoholic fatty liver disease. Aliment Pharmacol Ther 2010;32(3):487–97.
114. Cui X, You L, Zhu L, et al. Change in circulating microRNA profile of obese children indicates future risk of adult diabetes. Metabolism 2018;78:95–105.
115. Assmann TS, Riezu-Boj JI, Milagro FI, et al. Circulating adiposity-related microRNAs as predictors of the response to a low-fat diet in subjects with obesity. J Cell Mol Med 2020;24(5):2956–67.
116. Rossmeislová L, Mališová L, Kračmerová J, et al. Adaptation of human adipose tissue to hypocaloric diet. Int J Obes 2013;37(5):640–50.
117. Mariman ECM, Wang P. Adipocyte extracellular matrix composition, dynamics and role in obesity. Cell Mol Life Sci 2010;67(8):1277–92.
118. van Baak MA, Mariman ECM. Mechanisms of weight regain after weight loss — the role of adipose tissue. Nat Rev Endocrinol 2019;15(5):274–87.
119. Mutch DM, Pers TH, Temanni MR, et al. A distinct adipose tissue gene expression response to caloric restriction predicts 6-mo weight maintenance in obese subjects. Am J Clin Nutr 2011;94(6):1399–409.

120. Roumans NJT, Camps SG, Renes J, et al. Weight loss-induced stress in subcutaneous adipose tissue is related to weight regain. Br J Nutr 2016;115(5):913–20.
121. Roumans NJT, Vink RG, Gielen M, et al. Variation in extracellular matrix genes is associated with weight regain after weight loss in a sex-specific manner. Genes Nutr 2015;10(6):56.
122. Brummett BH, Babyak MA, Williams RB, et al. NEO personality domains and gender predict levels and trends in body mass index over 14 years during midlife. J Res Pers 2006;40(3):222–36.
123. Terracciano A, Sutin AR, McCrae RR, et al. Facets of personality linked to underweight and overweight. Psychosom Med 2009;71(6):682–9.
124. Kakizaki M, Kuriyama S, Sato Y, et al. Personality and body mass index: a cross-sectional analysis from the Miyagi Cohort Study. J Psychosom Res 2008;64(1):71–80.
125. Sutin AR, Ferrucci L, Zonderman AB, et al. Personality and obesity across the adult life span. J Pers Soc Psychol 2011;101(3):579–92.
126. Alkan A, Sahin I, Keskin L, et al. Diffusion-weighted imaging features of brain in obesity. Magn Reson Imaging 2008;26(4):446–50.
127. Mokhtari F, Rejeski WJ, Zhu Y, et al. Dynamic fMRI networks predict success in a behavioral weight loss program among older adults. Neuroimage 2018;173:421–33.
128. Istfan NW, Lipartia M, Anderson WA, et al. Approach to the Patient: Management of the Post-Bariatric Surgery Patient With Weight Regain. J Clin Endocrinol Metab 2021;106(1):251–63.
129. Goodarzi MO. Genetics of obesity: what genetic association studies have taught us about the biology of obesity and its complications. Lancet Diabetes Endocrinol 2018;6(3):223–36.
130. Yengo L, Sidorenko J, Kemper KE, et al. Meta-analysis of genome-wide association studies for height and body mass index in ~700000 individuals of European ancestry. Hum Mol Genet 2018;27(20):3641–9.
131. Reduction in the Incidence of Type 2 Diabetes with Lifestyle Intervention or Metformin. N Engl J Med 2002;346(6):393–403.
132. Look AHEAD Research Group, Pi-Sunyer X, Blackburn G, et al. Reduction in weight and cardiovascular disease risk factors in individuals with type 2 diabetes: one-year results of the look AHEAD trial. Diabetes Care 2007;30(6):1374–83.
133. Papandonatos GD, Pan Q, Pajewski NM, et al. Genetic Predisposition to Weight Loss and Regain With Lifestyle Intervention: Analyses From the Diabetes Prevention Program and the Look AHEAD Randomized Controlled Trials. Diabetes 2015;64(12):4312–21.
134. Delahanty LM, Pan Q, Jablonski KA, et al. Genetic predictors of weight loss and weight regain after intensive lifestyle modification, metformin treatment, or standard care in the Diabetes Prevention Program. Diabetes Care 2012;35(2):363–6.
135. McCaffery JM, Papandonatos GD, Huggins GS, et al. FTO predicts weight regain in the Look AHEAD clinical trial. Int J Obes 2013;37(12):1545–52.
136. Lewontin RC. The analysis of variance and the analysis of causes. 1974. Int J Epidemiol 2006;35(3):520–5.
137. Kolotkin RL, Crosby RD, Williams GR, et al. The relationship between health-related quality of life and weight loss. Obes Res 2001;9(9):564–71.

138. Wing RR, Lang W, Wadden TA, et al. Benefits of modest weight loss in improving cardiovascular risk factors in overweight and obese individuals with type 2 diabetes. Diabetes Care 2011;34(7):1481–6.
139. Haase CL, Lopes S, Olsen AH, et al. Weight loss and risk reduction of obesity-related outcomes in 0.5 million people: evidence from a UK primary care database. Int J Obes 2021;45(6):1249–58.
140. Sullivan M, Karlsson J, Sjöström L, et al. Swedish obese subjects (SOS)–an intervention study of obesity. Baseline evaluation of health and psychosocial functioning in the first 1743 subjects examined. Int J Obes Relat Metab Disord 1993;17(9):503–12. Available at: https://www.ncbi.nlm.nih.gov/pubmed/8220652.
141. Richards MM, Adams TD, Hunt SC. Functional status and emotional well-being, dietary intake, and physical activity of severely obese subjects. J Am Diet Assoc 2000;100(1):67–75.
142. Fine JT, Colditz GA, Coakley EH, et al. A prospective study of weight change and health-related quality of life in women. JAMA 1999;282(22):2136–42.
143. Engel SG, Crosby RD, Kolotkin RL, et al. Impact of weight loss and regain on quality of life: mirror image or differential effect? Obes Res 2003;11(10):1207–13.
144. Bogden JD, Kemp FW, Huang AE, et al. Bone mineral density and content during weight cycling in female rats: effects of dietary amylase-resistant starch. Nutr Metab 2008;5:34. https://doi.org/10.1186/1743-7075-5-34.
145. Anderson EK, Gutierrez DA, Kennedy A, et al. Weight cycling increases T-cell accumulation in adipose tissue and impairs systemic glucose tolerance. Diabetes 2013;62(9):3180–8.
146. Mehta T, Smith DL Jr, Muhammad J, et al. Impact of weight cycling on risk of morbidity and mortality. Obes Rev 2014;15(11):870–81.
147. King WC, Hinerman AS, Belle SH, et al. Comparison of the Performance of Common Measures of Weight Regain After Bariatric Surgery for Association With Clinical Outcomes. JAMA 2018;320(15):1560–9.

Management of Menopause Symptoms and Quality of Life during the Menopause Transition

Louie Ye, MD, PhD[a,b], Benita Knox, MD[a],
Martha Hickey, MBChB, MD[a,b,*]

KEYWORDS

- Menopause • Menopause-related quality of life • Vasomotor symptoms
- Urogenital symptoms

KEY POINTS

- Vasomotor and urogenital symptoms of menopause are associated with a physiologic decline in estrogen.
- Systemic menopausal hormone therapy improves vasomotor symptoms, and vaginal estrogen improves urogenital symptoms.
- Nonhormonal, non-pharmacologic options are also available.
- Neurokinin 3 receptor antagonist is a potential targeted therapy for vasomotor symptoms.
- Therapies should be evaluated for efficacy and impact on quality of life.

INTRODUCTION

Natural menopause is characterized by 12 months of amenorrhea without another established cause. It occurs at a median age of 51 years and is thought to reflect the depletion of the primordial follicle pool and reduction in ovarian estradiol production. Stages of menopause are described by the Stages of Reproductive Aging Workshop staging system: reproductive years, menopausal transition (perimenopause), and postmenopause.[1] Menopause that occurs between the age of 40 and 45 years or less than 40 years are referred to as early menopause and primary ovarian insufficiency (POI), respectively. Menopause can be iatrogenic, for example, via bilateral oophorectomy for the prevention or treatment of cancer or for benign indications. Both early menopause and POI have been associated with a range of adverse long-term

[a] The Royal Women's Hospital, 20 Flemington Road, Melbourne, Victoria 3052, Australia; [b] The Department of Obstetrics and Gynaecology, University of Melbourne and the Royal Women's Hospital, Lv 7 20 Flemington Road, Melbourne, Victoria 3052, Australia
* Corresponding author. The Department of Obstetrics and Gynaecology, University of Melbourne and the Royal Women's Hospital, Lv 7 20 Flemington Road, Melbourne, Victoria 3052.
E-mail address: hickeym@unimelb.edu.au

Endocrinol Metab Clin N Am 51 (2022) 817–836
https://doi.org/10.1016/j.ecl.2022.04.006
0889-8529/22/

outcomes. Menopause transition can vary in length and may be characterized by hot flashes or vasomotor symptoms (VMS), urogenital symptoms, sleep and mood disturbance, and joint/muscle pains. The prevalence and impact of these symptoms on women's quality of life globally have been subject to extensive investigations in recent years.[2] Menopause-related symptoms may influence health-related quality of life (HRQoL).[3] As a corollary, menopause-related or specific quality of life assessments (via tools such as the Menopause-Specific Quality of Life Questionnaire [MENQOL]) are important outcomes when assessing the impact of any intervention for menopausal symptoms, as they may inform clinicians and patients about the value of an intervention. Interventions for menopausal symptoms have continued to evolve.[4,5] This review provides an update focusing on the latest evidence-based and experimental approach for managing common symptoms (vasomotor, urogenital, sleep, and mood) to improve quality of life.[6]

VASOMOTOR SYMPTOMS

VMS, reported by 60% to 80% of women in the late menopausal transition to early postmenopausal stage, are characterized by a sudden sensation of heat in the face and chest.[7,8,9,10] Symptoms can last several minutes and occur from more than once every hour to less than once a day. Women who experience hot flashes at night-time may also report significant sleep disturbances.[11,12,13]

Non-pharmacologic Management

Most women experience mild VMS (ie, those that do not impact daily activities of living) and do not need or want pharmacotherapy. Evidence-based non-pharmacologic interventions recommended by professional bodies globally include cognitive-behavioral therapy (CBT) and hypnosis which have both shown efficacy in reducing VMS and improving sleep and mood disturbances (**Fig. 1**).[14,15,16,17,18,19,20,21,22,23] Primary care health professionals (ie, general practitioners and counselors) can facilitate CBT for VMS treatment over 4 to 6 weeks.[24,25] Recent evidence has also shown efficacy for telephone and Internet-based CBT to reduce the cost and improve the accessibility to treatment.[26,27,28,29] Similarly, hypnosis is another effective psychological treatment of VMS.[21,23] Hypnosis is a mind–body therapy that patients can practice (ie, self-hypnosis) as part of a self-help program as well as under the supervision of hypnosis practitioners.[30] Further studies are required to support the use of strategies such as diet/supplements, exercise, yoga, and acupuncture.[31]

Pharmacotherapy for Vasomotor Symptoms

Women who experience moderate-to-severe VMS may seek pharmacologic therapy. Historically, exogenous estrogen was recognized as the mainstay of VMS management until evidence emerged about risks published from the Women's Health Initiative studies.[32,33,34,35] In recent years, newer generations of hormonal and nonhormonal pharmacotherapy have been developed for the treatment of VMS.

Hormonal Pharmacotherapy Vasomotor Symptoms

Estrogen replacement, also known generically as menopause hormone therapy (MHT), describes both unopposed estrogen therapy (ET) for women who have undergone hysterectomy and combined estrogen–progestin therapy for women with an intact uterus, including both systemic and topical estrogen.[36] The efficacy of MHT in the management of vasomotor and urogenital symptoms is well-documented in contemporary literature. Overtime, MHT has evolved to include synthetic steroids

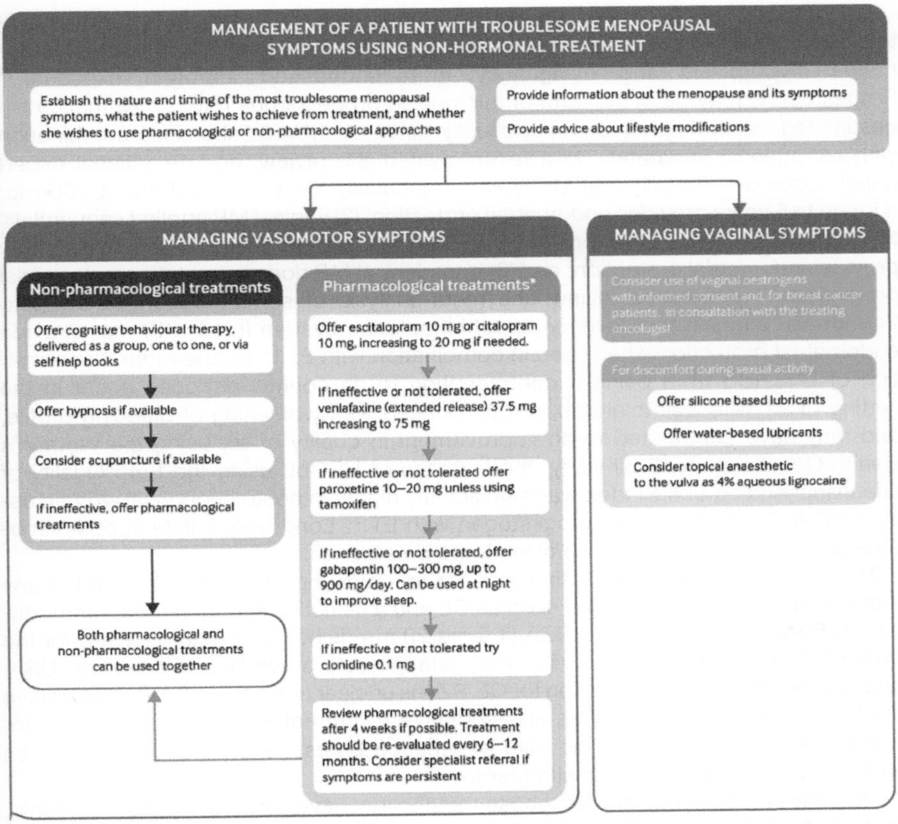

Fig. 1. Algorithm for using nonhormonal treatment of women with menopausal symptoms. (*Adapted from* Hickey M, Szabo RA, Hunter MS. Non-hormonal treatments for menopausal symptoms. BMJ. 2017 Nov 23;359:j5101.)

such as tibolone and other combined formulations such as conjugated equine estrogens and bazedoxifene (CE/BZA).[37] Several authors have published algorithms endorsed by professional bodies in recent years to facilitate the safe selection of an ever-growing list of hormonal therapies available for VMS.[4,5,38,39]

Although estrogen-based MHT may reduce VMS,[32,40] it does not prevent cardiovascular disease.[4] Of note, the US Preventive Service Task Force recently recommended against the use of combined estrogen and progestin for the primary prevention of chronic conditions in postmenopausal women.[41] Its use is associated with elevated risk for thromboembolic disease,[35,42] ischemic stroke,[42] breast cancer,[43,44,45,46] endometrial cancer,[47] ovarian cancer,[48] and gallbladder disease.[49,50]

Prescription choice for specific formulations is often based on theoretic efficacy—systemic oral estrogen such as 17-β estradiol is now more frequently used compared with CE due to its structural fidelity to ovarian-derived estrogen. Similarly, the route of administration is chosen based on woman's health profile—when systemic oral estrogen is contraindicated, transdermal estrogen is the recommended by several professional bodies, particularly for women who experience migraines with auras.[36,38,51,52,53]

Concomitant cyclical or continuous progestogen therapy is recommended for systemic MHT in all women who have not had a hysterectomy to reduce the risk of endometrial hyperplasia and malignancy from unopposed estrogen exposure.[54] Progestogens may be in the form of micronized progesterone (MP) or synthetic progestins (eg, medroxyprogesterone) usually taken orally in a fixed-dose combination with estrogen or separately. In a recent systematic review, an international expert panel concluded that (1) oral MP given sequentially for 12 to 14 d/mo at 200 mg/d for up to 5 years provides endometrial protection; (2) vaginal MP applied sequentially for 10 d/mo at 4% (45 mg/d) or every other day at 100 mg/d for up to 3 to 5 years may provide endometrial protection; and (3) transdermal MP does not provide endometrial protection. A systematic review and meta-analysis of six short-term trials (up to 24 months) suggest that levonorgestrel intrauterine system (LNG-IUS) may provide endometrial protection when used in combination with ET.[55] Furthermore, the transition of LNG-IUS from being a contraception to an counter-estrogen agent in the setting of ET was well tolerated, not associated with worsening of bleeding profile, and may have contributed to an improvement in quality of life using the Women's Health Questionnaire.[56] Similarly, the increase of HRQoL using the Euro Quality of Life Visual Analog Scale index was significantly higher in postmenopausal women using LNG-IUS compared oral progestogen with ET.[57] Long-term safety in postmenopausal women with LNG-IUS remains to be determined.

Tissue-selective estrogen complexes are an emerging class of hormonal therapy that consists of an oral estrogen such as CE and a selective estrogen receptor modulator (SERM) such as BZA. CE/BZA (4.5 mg/20 mg daily) is currently licensed for the treatment of postmenopausal VMS and osteoporosis prevention in Australia, USA, and Europe. The clinical indication for CE/BZA is unclear albeit a previous comparative study suggests it may serve as an alternative to current estrogen-based MHT for women experiencing VMS who also experience breast tenderness or for women who cannot tolerate oral progestin therapy.[58]

Tibolone is a synthetic steroid whose metabolites have estrogenic, progestogenic, and weak androgenic effects. It is licensed in Australia and Europe but not in the United States as an alternative to estrogen-based MHT for the treatment of VMS.[37,59,60,61] Recent systematic review of 46 RCTs concluded that tibolone is more effective than placebo but less effective than estrogen-based MHT in reducing VMS.[62] Furthermore, tibolone has been shown in RCTs to improve bone density, reduce fracture risk, and improve sexual dysfunction.[59,60,61,63] With regard to side effects and safety concerns, tibolone is associated with a higher rate of irregular bleeding than placebo but a lower rate than combined MHT. Notwithstanding the higher rate of irregular bleeding, it is not associated with an increase in the risk of endometrial hyperplasia or cancer compared with combined hormone treatment.[62,63,64,65] Nevertheless, owing to the higher rate of irregular bleeding, tibolone is generally not recommended for premenopausal women.[21] Furthermore, tibolone's association with breast cancer requires further investigations; currently, it is associated with a small increase in breast cancer recurrence and ischemic stroke in women greater than 65 years.[59,62,63,66]

Nonhormonal Pharmacotherapy for Vasomotor Symptoms

A range of nonhormonal pharmacotherapy is recognized by professional societies as effective for women experiencing VMS who are not candidates for MHT due to (1) medical contraindications, (2) resurgent symptoms after cessation of MHT, and (3) personal preference.[21,22,23,38] The list of nonhormonal agents includes selective serotonin reuptake inhibitors (SSRIs) (paroxetine, citalopram, and escitalopram), serotonin, and norepinephrine reuptake inhibitors (SNRIs) (venlafaxine, desvenlafaxine), antiepileptics (gabapentin, pregabalin), clonidine, and oxybutynin (see **Fig. 1**).

SSRIs and SNRIs are the most well-studied nonhormonal pharmacotherapy effective in reducing VMS.[67,68,69] They have been shown to be superior to placebo in a meta-analysis of 43 trials of nonhormonal therapies for VMS,[70] pooled analysis of seven RCTs of SSRIs/SNRIs,[71] and individual RCTs of SSRIs/SNRIs.[72,73,74,75,76,77,78,79] Furthermore, pooled analysis of 20 studies suggests that SSRIs and SNRIs are equally effective in women with breast cancer and in women with surgical or natural menopause.[80] Only venlafaxine has been reported to have similar efficacy for VMS as low-dose systemic estradiol.[81] Several limitations exist for SSRI/SNRIs as a therapy for VMS: (1) lack of longer-term data for safety and duration of efficacy after cessation and (2) no direct comparison of efficacy between various SSRIs/SNRIs.

Paroxetine and citalopram/escitalopram are well-studied SSRIs for the treatment of VMS with similar side effect profiles. Paroxetine is the only US Food and Drug Administration (FDA) approved SSRI for the treatment of VMS; it has been proposed as the first choice of SSRIs for its efficacy and FDA approval status.[82] Women treated with paroxetine reported a median reduction of 6.1 hot flashes per week with paroxetine compared with 2.8 with placebo. Reductions in hot flash frequency for this group range between 25% to 69% and 27% to 61% for hot flash severity.[83] Efficacy has been shown for paroxetine mesylate (7.5 mg/d) and paroxetine hydrochloride (10/20 mg day and 12.5/24 mg/d—controlled release).[73,76,82] Citalopram/escitalopram have been used at 20 mg daily with minimal side effects and significant improvement in menopause-related quality of life.[79,84,85,86,87]

Although paroxetine effectively reduces VMS, it may interfere with tamoxifen metabolism. Venlafaxine has minimal interaction with tamoxifen metabolism and is therefore the preferred SNRI for women taking tamoxifen. Studies have demonstrated 65% to 75% reductions in hot flashes compared with placebo and low doses of estradiol as well as a significant improvement in menopause-related quality of life.[81,88,89,90] Venlafaxine, however, has been reported to cause nausea/vomiting and significant withdrawal symptoms that may be reduced by the use of sustained-release formulation 37.5 mg 1 week before reaching a maintenance daily dose of 75 mg/d, with a similar step-down approach when planning cessation.[75] Similarly, desvenlafaxine (the main active metabolite of venlafaxine) at 100 mg daily can effectively reduce hot flashes albeit it shares similar side effect prolife as venlafaxine without the need for dose escalation.[91] Other reported side effects of antidepressants include nausea, dizziness, fatigue, sexual dysfunction, and rarely bone fracture and increased suicidal ideation in younger patients.[82] Contraindications to SSRIs and SNRIs include prior neuroleptic syndrome, serotonin syndrome, and the use of monoamine oxidase inhibitors.[23] There are no specific guides to the duration of use as is the case with MHT. Regular review to evaluate the benefits and side effects is essential. Clinicians should taper SSRIs and SNRIs as with any antidepressant to avoid the development of withdrawal symptoms. Switching to another class of medications (eg, anticonvulsants) is a reasonable option when SSRI/SNRI is ineffective or poorly tolerated.

Gabapentin and pregabalin are neuromodulator anticonvulsants licensed for the treatment of neuropathic pain. They have recently been recognized as potential alternatives to SSRI/SNRIs for the treatment of VMS. Recent RCTs have demonstrated gabapentin/pregabalin's efficacy for the treatment of hot flashes with 900 mg/d dosing and 300 mg/d, respectively.[71,92,93,94,95,96] At much higher doses of gabapentin (ie, 2400 mg/d), its efficacy for reduction of VMS is comparable to conjugated estrogen (0.625 mg) albeit with significant side effects including somnolence, headache, dizziness, and disorientation.[97] The sedating effect of gabapentin and VMS reduction may work synergistically, especially for women with hot flashes and sleep dysfunction where bedtime gabapentin may relieve the hot flashes that awaken patients from sleep.[4] Furthermore, similar efficacy in VMS reduction was demonstrated for pregabalin compared with placebo.[96]

Current evidence does not support the use of combination therapy using gabapentin with an SSRI/SNRI.[98] Other less commonly used agents such as clonidine (alpha-2 adrenergic agonist) and oxybutynin (anticholinergic) have shown efficacy for relief of VMS compared with placebo.[70,99,100] Of note, a recent RCT demonstrated oxybutynin (2.5–5 mg twice daily) significantly reduced the severity and frequency of hot flashes compared with placebo in women who were not candidates for estrogen-based therapy (ie, women who had breast cancer).[100] Furthermore, improvements were reported in most Hot Flashes Related Daily Interference Scale (HFRDIS) measures and in overall quality of life despite reporting more side effects (eg, dry mouth) compared with placebo.[100]

UROGENITAL SYMPTOMS

Few studies have reported on the prevalence of urogenital symptoms (eg, vaginal dryness), also known as genitourinary syndrome of menopause.[101] Recent Internet surveys and Day-to-Day Impact of Vaginal Aging questionnaires (a validated patient-reported outcome measurement tool) found that vaginal dryness may affect up to 85% of women over the age of 40 years, associated with dyspareunia, vaginal itching, and irritation.[102,103] The prevalence of vaginal dryness was reported to be 4% of women in early perimenopause, 21% in late perimenopause, and 47% 3 years after menopause using unvalidated questionnaires developed by Kaufert and Syrotuik.[104,105]

First-line therapy for mild urogenital symptoms often relies on nonhormonal vaginal moisturizers and lubricants to improve vaginal dryness and reduce dyspareunia (see **Fig. 1**).[10] There is conflicting evidence for the efficacy of vaginal moisturizers and lubricants for the treatment of urogenital symptoms compared with hormonal therapy, further studies are required to address this issue.[106]

Hormonal Therapy for Urogenital Symptoms

Topical vaginal estrogen alone is the preferred MHT for women with isolated urogenital symptoms of menopause (ie, vaginal dryness) that does not respond to moisturizers and lubricants.[10,21,107] Topical estrogen may be used to supplement systemic MHT for women with VMS where urogenital symptoms are inadequately treated by systemic MHT alone. A recent RCT using the MENQOL questionnaire found that vaginal estrogen modestly improved menopause-related quality of life and sexual function in postmenopausal women with moderate–severe urogenital symptoms.[108]

Topical estrogen is available in the form of tablet/capsule, pessary ring, and cream. The lowest systemic absorption of estrogen with clinical benefits for urogenital symptoms can be achieved by using standard regimens of 4 mcg or 10 mcg estradiol tablet or capsule as well as 7.5 mcg/d estradiol ring.[109,110,111] Low-dose vaginal estrogen has not been linked to an increased risk of endometrial hyperplasia, neoplasia,[112,113] venous thromboembolism, breast cancer, or cardiovascular disease.[114,115,116] However, no studies have examined the impact of low-dose estrogen on the endometrium beyond the first year of treatment. There is some evidence of systemic absorption of topical estrogen at higher doses, with higher estradiol levels found in some women using this than would be expected in postmenopausal women.[117,118,119] Pessary rings or cream may reach premenopausal serum estradiol leading to endometrial proliferation.[111,120,121] Based on limited evidence and expert opinion, the use of a continuous progestin regimen is currently not recommended for women on low-dose vaginal estrogen, albeit women at risk of endometrial cancer may require endometrial surveillance (eg, transvaginal ultrasound) and intermittent progestin therapy.[122]

For treatment of dyspareunia in the setting of vulvovaginal atrophy, ospemifene is an SERM and an FDA-approved option for women who cannot or prefer not to use vaginal estrogen. Its efficacy (60 mg/d) over 12 weeks has been to reduce the severity of dyspareunia and vaginal dryness in several RCTs compared with placebo using the most bothersome symptoms scale, as well as an improvement in female sexual dysfunction using a well validated female sexual function index (FSFI) questionnaire, although direct comparisons are yet to be made against vaginal ET.[123,124,125,126] The most common side effect of ospemifene is hot flashes compared with placebo.[124] Serious adverse effects such as endometrial hyperplasia or carcinoma or thrombotic events require further investigations.[127]

Other options include vaginal dehydroepiandrosterone (DHEA) or prasterone (FDA approved vaginal suppository 6.5 mg/d) and tibolone. DHEA has also been shown to be effective for the treatment of dyspareunia and overall improvement in sexual function using the FSFI questionnaire in the setting of vulvovaginal atrophy secondary to menopause.[128,129,130] Similarly, women who received tibolone therapy experienced significant improvement in vaginal dryness, dyspareunia, and urinary symptoms.[131]

Non-pharmacologic Therapy for Urogenital Symptoms

Laser and radiofrequency devices have been developed for the treatment of vulvovaginal atrophy. Laser or radiofrequency energy is directed at vaginal wall tissue over several treatment sessions to remodel vaginal connective tissue.[132] A limited number of RCTs exist for laser treatment of urogenital symptoms with conflicting data for its efficacy.[133,134,135] A recent sham-controlled trial of vaginal laser did not find any improvement in vaginal symptoms after 12 months.[133] For now, laser or energy-based devices are neither endorsed nor approved by professional or regulatory bodies.[21,136,137]

SLEEP DISTURBANCE

Sleep disturbance or insomnia is a widely reported symptom beginning around menopausal transition, affecting up to 56% by postmenopause.[138] Sleep disturbance is classified into three groups: (1) trouble falling asleep, (2) multiple awakenings, and (3) waking up early.[139] Nocturnal awakening has been identified as one of the most common sleep disturbances and is associated with VMS.[139,140] Sleep disturbance during perimenopause can occur independently of VMS.[141] In a recent systematic review and meta-analysis, MHT has been shown to improve sleep quality in women with concurrent night-time VMS albeit independent effects of MHT on sleep disturbance require further evaluation.[142] Other forms of MHT such as CE/BZA have also been shown to significantly improve sleep quality, the time taken to fall asleep and the menopause-related quality of life, as assessed by the MENQOL and Medical Outcome Study (MOS) sleep scale.[143] Nonhormonal therapies such as SSRIs/SNRIs have not been evaluated to treat sleep disturbance alone but can be useful in women experiencing VMS with a concurrent mood disorder or sleep issues based on pooled analysis using the Insomnia Severity Index (ISI).[14,79] Similarly, the nonhormonal agent gabapentin has been shown to improve sleep quality in perimenopausal women with VMS and insomnia using the Pittsburgh Sleep Quality Index (PSQI)—a self-report questionnaire for the assessment of sleep quality.[144] Unfortunately, none of the aforementioned scales (MOS, ISI, and PSQI) have been validated in menopausal women. PSQI, however, has been identified to include the most relevant domains of sleep quality across many self-reported sleep scales in previous studies but a screening tool with sufficient domains of sleep quality that is validated in menopausal women remains to be developed.[142]

MOOD DISTURBANCE

Most women in menopausal transition do not develop new-onset major depressive disorder (MDD) but are at risk of developing depressive symptoms associated VMS and sleep disturbance.[145,146] Most women with depressive symptoms remain stable, about 9% of women experience increasing symptoms whereas another 8.5% experience decreasing symptoms.[147] Risk factors for increasing depressive symptoms include the previous history of depression, a history of hysterectomy plus oophorectomy, or prior cessation then resuming MHT.[147,148] Antidepressants and CBT remain the first-line treatment of depressive symptoms for perimenopausal women.[149] A previous history of MDD and the use of SSRI/SNRI would guide agent choice and dosing in perimenopause. To date, desvenlafaxine is the only antidepressant that has been studied in large RCTs of well-defined perimenopausal and postmenopausal women with MDD showing efficacy in reduction of depressive symptoms compared with placebo using the Hamilton Depression Rating Scale—the "gold standard" assessment of severity as well as change in depressive symptoms.[150,151] Another instrument most commonly used to assess mood during menopause is the Center of Epidemiologic Studies Depression Scale—a self-report depression screening tool designed for symptoms of depressed mood in older adults, validated across a range of ages albeit not specifically in menopausal women.[152] Furthermore, current evidence is insufficient for recommending MHT or herbal remedies for menopause-related depressive symptoms.[148]

NEW DEVELOPMENTS IN TARGETED THERAPY

In recent years, unregulated activation of kisspeptin/neurokinin B/dynorphin (KNDy) expressing neurons by neurokinin B (NKB) has been implicated in the development of VMS. KNDy neurons reside in the thermoregulatory center in the hypothalamus and are stimulated by NKB and inhibited by estrogen (**Fig. 2**). With the decline of estrogen during menopause, NKB signaling becomes unregulated leading to unopposed KNDy activation resulting in VMS.[153,154,155] Inhibition of the NKB signaling at its receptor (neurokinin 3 receptor [NK3R]) has been tested as a therapy to reduce KNDy neuron activation. The efficacy of a NK3R antagonist was previously demonstrated in a phase 2 RCT. An oral NK3R antagonist (MLE4901) reduced hot flashes per day by 45% and improved quality-of-life domains as assessed by validated outcome tools such as HFRDIS and MENQOL questionnaires.[156] A similar reduction of hot flashes and improvement in quality-of-life domains was reported with an alternative oral NK3R antagonist (fezolinetant) using a range of validated outcome tools including HFRDIS, Leeds Sleep Evaluation Questionnaire, Greene Climacteric Scale, and Sheehan Disability Scale.[157,158,159] Adverse effects noted in these early studies include drug-induced transient transaminitis, but more commonly, nausea, diarrhea, headache, and cough.[156,157] Larger scale studies of longer duration are required before clinical implementation.

NEW DEVELOPMENTS IN TRIAL DESIGNS

To improve the consistency of outcome measures, future studies evaluating the safety and efficacy of treatments for VMS and urogenital symptoms should examine

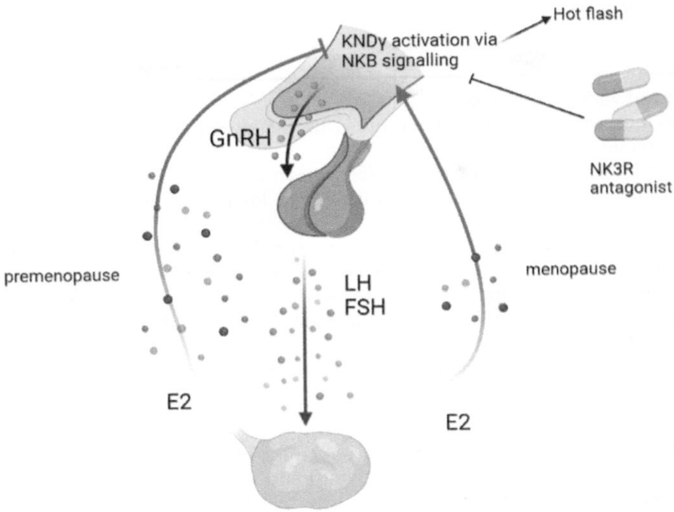

Fig. 2. Theoretic physiologic changes in neurohormonal pathways involved in the development of hot flashes and the role of NK3R antagonist. Premenopause estrogen level (left of HPO axis) inhibits KNDy neuron activation thereby development of hot flashes. With the reduction in estrogen level in menopause (right of HPO axis), KNDy neurons become less inhibited leading to hot flashes. NK3R antagonist may reduce KNDy neuron activation thereby reducing hot flashes. E2, estrogen; FSH, follicle-stimulating hormone; GnRH, gonadotrophin-releasing hormone; LH, luteinizing hormone; HPO, hypothalamiic ovarian axis.

outcomes that are most important to symptomatic women. Core outcome set (COS) has recently been developed for use in clinical trials of treatments for VMS and urogenital symptoms.[160,161] With regard to VMS COS, the six outcomes include (1) frequency of VMS, (2) severity of VMS, (3) distress, bother, or inference caused by VMS, (4) impact on sleep, (5) satisfaction with treatment, and (6) side effects of treatment.[160] With regard to urogenital symptoms associated with menopause, the final COS includes eight outcomes: (1) pain with sex; (2) vulvovaginal dryness; (3) vulvovaginal discomfort or irritation; (4) discomfort or pain when urinating: (5) change in most bothersome symptom: (6) distress, bother, or interference of genitourinary symptoms; (7) satisfaction with treatment; and (8) side effects of treatment.[161] The implementation of these COSs will not only capture the priorities for women, clinicians, and researchers but also standardize outcome reporting which will allow meaningful comparisons of results from different studies, ultimately improving outcomes for women with VMS and urogenital symptoms.

SUMMARY

For some women, menopause can be associated with bothersome symptoms that impact their quality of life and lead them to seek information or treatment. Although MHT was historically the treatment of choice for menopausal symptoms, medical contraindications and personal preference for nonhormonal therapy have created an impetus to identify safer alternative therapies for the treatment of the common symptoms of menopause. Much work remains to be done to optimize existing therapies and discover new therapies with an emphasis on each treatment's impact on quality of life.

CLINICS CARE POINTS[a]

Management of vasomotor symptoms (VMS)

- Prescribers must individualize care and prescribe the lowest effective dose for the shortest duration needed to relieve VMS
- Estrogen only therapy can be prescribed for women who have undergone hysterectomy
- Combination of estrogen and progestin is needed for women who have not undergone hysterectomy
- Women with premature or early menopause should be offered menopause hormone therapy (MHT) at least until the age of 50 years unless otherwise contraindicated
- Cognitive-behavioral therapy or selective serotonin reuptake inhibitor/serotonin and norepinephrine reuptake inhibitor/clonidine/gabapentin should be offered for the treatment of VMS if MHT is not suitable
- Paroxetine and fluoxetine should be avoided in women taking tamoxifen
- MHT should not be prescribed for the prevention of chronic disease

Management of urogenital symptoms

- Consider lubricants with sexual activity and regular use of long-acting vaginal moisturizers as the first-line treatment of mild urogenital symptoms
- Low-dose vaginal estrogen therapy (ET) is effective for the management of urogenital symptoms. Systemic ET can be used when VMS are present; consider vaginal dehydroepiandrosterone or ospemifene if symptoms unresponsive to first-line therapy

Inform and Refer

- Women who are concerned about cardiovascular disease risks of MHT should be informed that MHT use within 10 years of menopause does not seem to increase the risk of coronary heart disease
- Consider mental health referral in women with symptoms of mood disorder and women with a history of affective disorders
- Consider appropriate specialist referrals for women undergoing premature/surgical menopause or following a cancer diagnosis

[a]Based on various society guidelines (Level A evidence) including recommendations from NAMS, American College of Obstetrics and Gynecology (ACOG), and Royal Australia and New Zealand College of Obstetrics and Gynaecology (RANZCOG).

ACKNOWLEDGMENTS

Martha Hickey is funded by a National Health and Medical Research Council Investigator Grant (L2).

DISCLOSURE

The authors of this review do not have any commercial or financial conflicts of interest and/or any funding sources.

REFERENCES

1. Harlow SD, Gass M, Hall JE, et al. Executive summary of the stages of reproductive aging workshop + 10: addressing the unfinished agenda of staging reproductive aging. Menopause 2012;19(4):387–95.
2. Palacios S. Prevalence and impact on quality of life of vasomotor symptoms. Menopause 2021;28(8):850–1.
3. Blumel JE, Castelo-Branco C, Binfa L, et al. Quality of life after the menopause: a population study. Maturitas 2000;34(1):17–23.

4. Santoro N, Roeca C, Peters BA, et al. The Menopause transition: signs, symptoms, and management options. J Clin Endocrinol Metab 2021;106(1):1–15.
5. Santoro N, Epperson CN, Mathews SB. Menopausal symptoms and their management. Endocrinol Metab Clin North Am 2015;44(3):497–515.
6. Proceedings from the NIH State-of-the-Science Conference on Management of Menopause-Related Symptoms, March 21-23, 2005, Bethesda, Maryland, USA. Am J Med 2005;118(Suppl 12B):1–171.
7. Thurston RC, Joffe H. Vasomotor symptoms and menopause: findings from the Study of Women's Health across the Nation. Obstet Gynecol Clin North Am 2011;38(3):489–501.
8. McKinlay SM, Brambilla DJ, Posner JG. The normal menopause transition. Am J Hum Biol 1992;4(1):37–46.
9. McKinlay SM. The normal menopause transition: an overview. Maturitas 1996; 23(2):137–45.
10. ACOG Practice Bulletin No. 141: management of menopausal symptoms. Obstet Gynecol 2014;123(1):202–16.
11. Freedman RR, Roehrs TA. Effects of REM sleep and ambient temperature on hot flash-induced sleep disturbance. Menopause 2006;13(4):576–83.
12. Ohayon MM. Severe hot flashes are associated with chronic insomnia. Arch Intern Med 2006;166(12):1262–8.
13. Erlik Y, Tataryn IV, Meldrum DR, et al. Association of waking episodes with menopausal hot flushes. JAMA 1981;245(17):1741–4.
14. Guthrie KA, Larson JC, Ensrud KE, et al. Effects of Pharmacologic and Nonpharmacologic Interventions on Insomnia Symptoms and Self-reported Sleep Quality in Women With Hot Flashes: a Pooled Analysis of Individual Participant Data From Four MsFLASH Trials. Sleep 2018;41(1).
15. Green SM, Donegan E, Frey BN, et al. Cognitive behavior therapy for menopausal symptoms (CBT-Meno): a randomized controlled trial. Menopause 2019;26(9):972–80.
16. Mann E, Smith MJ, Hellier J, et al. Cognitive behavioural treatment for women who have menopausal symptoms after breast cancer treatment (MENOS 1): a randomised controlled trial. Lancet Oncol 2012;13(3):309–18.
17. Tao WW, Tao XM, Song CL. Effects of non-pharmacological supportive care for hot flushes in breast cancer: a meta-analysis. Support Care Cancer 2017;25(7): 2335–47.
18. Elkins G. Behavioral interventions for hot flashes. Menopause 2013;20(12):1312.
19. Elkins G, Marcus J, Stearns V, et al. Randomized trial of a hypnosis intervention for treatment of hot flashes among breast cancer survivors. J Clin Oncol 2008; 26(31):5022–6.
20. Cramer H, Lauche R, Paul A, et al. Hypnosis in breast cancer care: a systematic review of randomized controlled trials. Integr Cancer Ther 2015;14(1):5–15.
21. RANZCOG. Managing menopausal symptoms. 2020. Available at: https://ranzcog.edu.au/RANZCOG_SITE/media/RANZCOG-MEDIA/Women%27s%20Health/Statement%20and%20guidelines/Clinical%20-%20Gynaecology/Managing-Menopausal-Symptoms-(C-Gyn-9)_September-2020.pdf?ext=.pdf. Accessed May 2021.
22. NICE. Menopause: diagnosis and management. 2019. Available at: https://www.nice.org.uk/guidance/ng23/resources/menopause-diagnosis-and-management-pdf-1837330217413. Accessed May 2021.
23. Carpenter J, Gass MLS, Maki PM, et al. Nonhormonal management of menopause-associated vasomotor symptoms: 2015 position statement of The

North American Menopause Society. Menopause-The J North Am Menopause Soc 2015;22(11):1155–74.
24. Hunter M, Smith M. Managing hot flushes with group cognitive behaviour therapy : an evidence based treatment manual for health professionals. London ; New York: Routledge, a Taylor & Francis Group; 2015.
25. Hunter M, Smith M. In: Park Milton, Abingdon, editors. Managing hot flushes and night sweats : a cognitive behavioural self-help guide to the menopause. Second edition. Oxon ; New York, NY: Routledge; 2021.
26. Atema V, van Leeuwen M, Kieffer JM, et al. Internet-based cognitive behavioral therapy aimed at alleviating treatment-induced menopausal symptoms in breast cancer survivors: Moderators and mediators of treatment effects. Maturitas 2020;131:8–13.
27. Verbeek JGE, Atema V, Mewes JC, et al. Cost-utility, cost-effectiveness, and budget impact of Internet-based cognitive behavioral therapy for breast cancer survivors with treatment-induced menopausal symptoms. Breast Cancer Res Treat 2019;178(3):573–85.
28. Atema V, van Leeuwen M, Kieffer JM, et al. Efficacy of Internet-Based Cognitive Behavioral Therapy for Treatment-Induced Menopausal Symptoms in Breast Cancer Survivors: Results of a Randomized Controlled Trial. J Clin Oncol 2019;37(10):809–22.
29. McCurry SM, Guthrie KA, Morin CM, et al. Telephone-Based Cognitive Behavioral Therapy for Insomnia in Perimenopausal and Postmenopausal Women With Vasomotor Symptoms: A MsFLASH Randomized Clinical Trial. JAMA Intern Med 2016;176(7):913–20.
30. Elkins GR. Relief from hot flashes : the natural, drug-free program to reduce hot flashes, improve sleep, and ease stress. New York: demosHealth, LLC; 2014.
31. McCormick CA, Brennan A, Hickey M. Managing vasomotor symptoms effectively without hormones. Climacteric 2020;23(6):532–8.
32. Barnabei VM, Cochrane BB, Aragaki AK, et al. Menopausal symptoms and treatment-related effects of estrogen and progestin in the Women's Health Initiative. Obstet Gynecol 2005;105(5 Pt 1):1063–73.
33. Crawford SL, Crandall CJ, Derby CA, et al. Menopausal hormone therapy trends before versus after 2002: impact of the Women's Health Initiative Study Results. Menopause 2018;26(6):588–97.
34. DeNeui T, Berg J, Howson A. Best practices in care for menopausal patients: 16 years after the Women's Health Initiative. J Am Assoc Nurse Pract 2019;31(7):420–7.
35. Manson JE, Chlebowski RT, Stefanick ML, et al. Menopausal hormone therapy and health outcomes during the intervention and extended poststopping phases of the Women's Health Initiative randomized trials. JAMA 2013;310(13):1353–68.
36. The NHTPSAP. The 2017 hormone therapy position statement of The North American Menopause Society. Menopause 2017;24(7):728–53.
37. de Villiers TJ, Hall JE, Pinkerton JV, et al. Revised global consensus statement on menopausal hormone therapy. Maturitas 2016;91:153–5.
38. Stuenkel CA, Davis SR, Gompel A, et al. Treatment of Symptoms of the Menopause: An Endocrine Society Clinical Practice Guideline. J Clin Endocrinol Metab 2015;100(11):3975–4011.
39. Jane FM, Davis SR. A practitioner's toolkit for managing the menopause. Climacteric 2014;17(5):564–79.

40. Hulley S, Grady D, Bush T, et al. Randomized trial of estrogen plus progestin for secondary prevention of coronary heart disease in postmenopausal women. Heart and Estrogen/progestin Replacement Study (HERS) Research Group. JAMA 1998;280(7):605–13.
41. Force USPST, Grossman DC, Curry SJ, et al. Hormone Therapy for the Primary Prevention of Chronic Conditions in Postmenopausal Women: US Preventive Services Task Force Recommendation Statement. JAMA 2017;318(22): 2224–33.
42. Rovinski D, Ramos RB, Fighera TM, et al. Risk of venous thromboembolism events in postmenopausal women using oral versus non-oral hormone therapy: a systematic review and meta-analysis. Thromb Res 2018;168:83–95.
43. Anderson GL, Limacher M, Assaf AR, et al. Effects of conjugated equine estrogen in postmenopausal women with hysterectomy: the Women's Health Initiative randomized controlled trial. JAMA 2004;291(14):1701–12.
44. Rossouw JE, Anderson GL, Prentice RL, et al. Risks and benefits of estrogen plus progestin in healthy postmenopausal women: principal results From the Women's Health Initiative randomized controlled trial. JAMA 2002;288(3): 321–33.
45. Collaborative Group on Hormonal Factors in Breast C. Type and timing of menopausal hormone therapy and breast cancer risk: individual participant meta-analysis of the worldwide epidemiological evidence. Lancet 2019;394(10204): 1159–68.
46. Chlebowski RT, Hendrix SL, Langer RD, et al. Influence of estrogen plus progestin on breast cancer and mammography in healthy postmenopausal women: the Women's Health Initiative Randomized Trial. JAMA 2003;289(24):3243–53.
47. Allen NE, Tsilidis KK, Key TJ, et al. Menopausal hormone therapy and risk of endometrial carcinoma among postmenopausal women in the European Prospective Investigation Into Cancer and Nutrition. Am J Epidemiol 2010; 172(12):1394–403.
48. Beral V, Gaitskell K, Hermon C, et al, Collaborative Group On Epidemiological Studies Of Ovarian C. Menopausal hormone use and ovarian cancer risk: individual participant meta-analysis of 52 epidemiological studies. Lancet 2015; 385(9980):1835–42.
49. Cirillo DJ, Wallace RB, Rodabough RJ, et al. Effect of estrogen therapy on gallbladder disease. JAMA 2005;293(3):330–9.
50. Simon JA, Hunninghake DB, Agarwal SK, et al. Effect of estrogen plus progestin on risk for biliary tract surgery in postmenopausal women with coronary artery disease. The Heart and Estrogen/progestin Replacement Study. Ann Intern Med 2001;135(7):493–501.
51. North American Menopause S. The 2012 hormone therapy position statement of: The North American Menopause Society. Menopause 2012;19(3):257–71.
52. Santen RJ, Allred DC, Ardoin SP, et al. Postmenopausal hormone therapy: an Endocrine Society scientific statement. J Clin Endocrinol Metab 2010;95(7 Suppl 1):s1–66.
53. Shifren JL, Schiff I. Role of hormone therapy in the management of menopause. Obstet Gynecol 2010;115(4):839–55.
54. Effects of hormone replacement therapy on endometrial histology in postmenopausal women. The Postmenopausal Estrogen/Progestin Interventions (PEPI) Trial. The Writing Group for the PEPI Trial. JAMA 1996;275(5):370–5.
55. Somboonporn W, Panna S, Temtanakitpaisan T, et al. Effects of the levonorgestrel-releasing intrauterine system plus estrogen therapy in

perimenopausal and postmenopausal women: systematic review and meta-analysis. Menopause 2011;18(10):1060–6.
56. Depypere HT, Hillard T, Erkkola R, et al. A 60-month non-comparative study on bleeding profiles with the levonorgestrel intrauterine system from the late transition period to estrogen supplemented menopause. Eur J Obstet Gynecol Reprod Biol 2010;153(2):176–80.
57. Pirimoglu ZM, Ozyapi AG, Kars B, et al. Comparing the effects of intrauterine progestin system and oral progestin on health-related quality of life and Kupperman index in hormone replacement therapy. J Obstet Gynaecol Res 2011; 37(10):1376–81.
58. Pinkerton JV, Harvey JA, Pan K, et al. Breast effects of bazedoxifene-conjugated estrogens: a randomized controlled trial. Obstet Gynecol 2013;121(5):959–68.
59. Huang KE, Baber R. Asia Pacific Tibolone Consensus G. Updated clinical recommendations for the use of tibolone in Asian women. Climacteric 2010;13(4): 317–27.
60. Nathorst-Boos J, Hammar M. Effect on sexual life–a comparison between tibolone and a continuous estradiol-norethisterone acetate regimen. Maturitas 1997; 26(1):15–20.
61. Kokcu A, Cetinkaya MB, Yanik F, et al. The comparison of effects of tibolone and conjugated estrogen-medroxyprogesterone acetate therapy on sexual performance in postmenopausal women. Maturitas 2000;36(1):75–80.
62. Formoso G, Perrone E, Maltoni S, et al. Short-term and long-term effects of tibolone in postmenopausal women. Cochrane Database Syst Rev 2016;10(10): CD008536.
63. Cummings SR, Ettinger B, Delmas PD, et al. The effects of tibolone in older postmenopausal women. N Engl J Med 2008;359(7):697–708.
64. Hammar ML, van de Weijer P, Franke HR, et al. Tibolone and low-dose continuous combined hormone treatment: vaginal bleeding pattern, efficacy and tolerability. BJOG 2007;114(12):1522–9.
65. Archer DF, Hendrix S, Gallagher JC, et al. Endometrial effects of tibolone. J Clin Endocrinol Metab 2007;92(3):911–8.
66. Kenemans P, Bundred NJ, Foidart JM, et al. Safety and efficacy of tibolone in breast-cancer patients with vasomotor symptoms: a double-blind, randomised, non-inferiority trial. Lancet Oncol 2009;10(2):135–46.
67. Rada G, Capurro D, Pantoja T, et al. Non-hormonal interventions for hot flushes in women with a history of breast cancer. Cochrane Database Syst Rev 2010;(9): CD004923.
68. Sideras K, Loprinzi CL. Nonhormonal management of hot flashes for women on risk reduction therapy. J Natl Compr Canc Netw 2010;8(10):1171–9.
69. Shams T, Firwana B, Habib F, et al. SSRIs for hot flashes: a systematic review and meta-analysis of randomized trials. J Gen Intern Med 2014;29(1):204.
70. Nelson HD, Vesco KK, Haney E, et al. Nonhormonal therapies for menopausal hot flashes: systematic review and meta-analysis. JAMA 2006;295(17):2057–71.
71. Loprinzi CL, Sloan J, Stearns V, et al. Newer antidepressants and gabapentin for hot flashes: an individual patient pooled analysis. J Clin Oncol 2009;27(17): 2831–7.
72. Loprinzi CL, Kugler JW, Sloan JA, et al. Venlafaxine in management of hot flashes in survivors of breast cancer: a randomised controlled trial. Lancet 2000;356(9247):2059–63.

73. Stearns V, Beebe KL, Iyengar M, et al. Paroxetine controlled release in the treatment of menopausal hot flashes: a randomized controlled trial. JAMA 2003; 289(21):2827–34.
74. Loprinzi CL, Sloan JA, Perez EA, et al. Phase III evaluation of fluoxetine for treatment of hot flashes. J Clin Oncol 2002;20(6):1578–83.
75. Evans ML, Pritts E, Vittinghoff E, et al. Management of postmenopausal hot flushes with venlafaxine hydrochloride: a randomized, controlled trial. Obstet Gynecol 2005;105(1):161–6.
76. Stearns V, Slack R, Greep N, et al. Paroxetine is an effective treatment for hot flashes: results from a prospective randomized clinical trial. J Clin Oncol 2005;23(28):6919–30.
77. Loprinzi CL, Barton DL, Sloan JA, et al. Mayo Clinic and North Central Cancer Treatment Group hot flash studies: a 20-year experience. Menopause 2008; 15(4 Pt 1):655–60.
78. Barton DL, LaVasseur BI, Sloan JA, et al. Phase III, placebo-controlled trial of three doses of citalopram for the treatment of hot flashes: NCCTG trial N05C9. J Clin Oncol 2010;28(20):3278–83.
79. Freeman EW, Guthrie KA, Caan B, et al. Efficacy of escitalopram for hot flashes in healthy menopausal women: a randomized controlled trial. JAMA 2011; 305(3):267–74.
80. Bardia A, Novotny P, Sloan J, et al. Efficacy of nonestrogenic hot flash therapies among women stratified by breast cancer history and tamoxifen use: a pooled analysis. Menopause 2009;16(3):477–83.
81. Joffe H, Guthrie KA, LaCroix AZ, et al. Low-dose estradiol and the serotonin-norepinephrine reuptake inhibitor venlafaxine for vasomotor symptoms: a randomized clinical trial. JAMA Intern Med 2014;174(7):1058–66.
82. Simon JA, Portman DJ, Kaunitz AM, et al. Low-dose paroxetine 7.5 mg for menopausal vasomotor symptoms: two randomized controlled trials. Menopause 2013;20(10):1027–35.
83. Soares CN, Joffe H, Viguera AC, et al. Paroxetine versus placebo for women in midlife after hormone therapy discontinuation. Am J Med 2008;121(2): 159-U112.
84. Barton DL, LaVasseur BI, Sloan JA. Phase III, placebo-controlled trial of three doses of citalopram for the treatment of hot flashes: NCCTG trial N05C9Vol 28. United States: American Society of Clinical Oncology; 2010. p. 3278–83.
85. LaCroix AZ, Freeman EW, Larson J, et al. Effects of escitalopram on menopause-specific quality of life and pain in healthy menopausal women with hot flashes: a randomized controlled trial. Maturitas 2012;73(4):361–8.
86. Kalay AE, Demir B, Haberal A, et al. Efficacy of citalopram on climacteric symptoms. Menopause 2007;14(2):223–9.
87. Suvanto-Luukkonen E, Koivunen R, Sundstrom H, et al. Citalopram and fluoxetine in the treatment of postmenopausal symptoms: a prospective, randomized, 9-month, placebo-controlled, double-blind study. Menopause 2005;12(1): 18–26.
88. Pinkerton JV, Joffe H, Kazempour K, et al. Low-dose paroxetine (7.5 mg) improves sleep in women with vasomotor symptoms associated with menopause. Menopause 2015;22(1):50–8.
89. Pinkerton JV, Constantine G, Hwang E, et al. Desvenlafaxine compared with placebo for treatment of menopausal vasomotor symptoms: a 12-week, multicenter, parallel-group, randomized, double-blind, placebo-controlled efficacy trial. Menopause 2013;20(1):28–37.

90. Caan B, LaCroix AZ, Joffe H, et al. Effects of estrogen and venlafaxine on menopause-related quality of life in healthy postmenopausal women with hot flashes: a placebo-controlled randomized trial. Menopause 2015;22(6):607–15.
91. Sperrof L, Gass, M, Constantine, G Obstet Gynecol.Efficacy and tolerability of desvenlafaxine succinate treatment for menopausal vasomotor symptoms: a randomized controlled trial 2008 Jan;111(1):77–7. https://doi.org/10.1097/01.AOG.0000297371.89129.b3.
92. Guttuso T Jr, Kurlan R, McDermott MP, et al. Gabapentin's effects on hot flashes in postmenopausal women: a randomized controlled trial. Obstet Gynecol 2003;101(2):337–45.
93. Pandya KJ, Morrow GR, Roscoe JA, et al. Gabapentin for hot flashes in 420 women with breast cancer: a randomised double-blind placebo-controlled trial. Lancet 2005;366(9488):818–24.
94. Loprinzi L, Barton DL, Sloan JA, et al. Pilot evaluation of gabapentin for treating hot flashes. Mayo Clin Proc 2002;77(11):1159–63.
95. Fitzpatrick LA, Santen RJ. Hot flashes: the old and the new, what is really true? Mayo Clin Proc 2002;77(11):1155–8.
96. Loprinzi CL, Qin R, Balcueva EP. Phase III, randomized, double-blind, placebo-controlled evaluation of pregabalin for alleviating hot flashes. J Clin Oncol 2010 Feb 1;28(4):641–7. https://doi.org/10.1200/JCO.2009.24.5647. Epub 2009 Nov 9.PMID: 19901102.
97. Reddy SY, Warner H, Guttuso T Jr, et al. Gabapentin, estrogen, and placebo for treating hot flushes: a randomized controlled trial. Obstet Gynecol 2006;108(1):41–8.
98. Loprinzi CL, Kugler JW, Barton DL, et al. Phase III trial of gabapentin alone or in conjunction with an antidepressant in the management of hot flashes in women who have inadequate control with an antidepressant alone: NCCTG N03C5. J Clin Oncol 2007;25(3):308–12.
99. Simon JA, Gaines T, LaGuardia KD. Extended-release oxybutynin therapy for vasomotor symptoms in women: a randomized clinical trial. Menopause 2016;23(11):1214–21.
100. Leon-Ferre RA, Novotny PJ, Wolfe EG, et al. Oxybutynin vs Placebo for Hot Flashes in Women With or Without Breast Cancer: A Randomized, Double-Blind Clinical Trial (ACCRU SC-1603). JNCI Cancer Spectr 2020;4(1):pkz088.
101. Portman DJ, Gass ML. Vulvovaginal Atrophy Terminology Consensus Conference P. Genitourinary syndrome of menopause: new terminology for vulvovaginal atrophy from the International Society for the Study of Women's Sexual Health and the North American Menopause Society. Maturitas 2014;79(3):349–54.
102. Huang AJ, Gregorich SE, Kuppermann M, et al. Day-to-Day Impact of Vaginal Aging questionnaire: a multidimensional measure of the impact of vaginal symptoms on functioning and well-being in postmenopausal women. Menopause 2015;22(2):144–54.
103. Krychman M, Graham S, Bernick B, et al. The Women's EMPOWER Survey: Women's Knowledge and Awareness of Treatment Options for Vulvar and Vaginal Atrophy Remains Inadequate. J Sex Med 2017;14(3):425–33.
104. Dennerstein L, Dudley EC, Hopper JL, et al. A prospective population-based study of menopausal symptoms. Obstet Gynecol 2000;96(3):351–8.
105. Kaufert P, Syrotuik J. Symptom reporting at the menopause. Soc Sci Med E 1981;15(3):173–84.

106. Mitchell CM, Reed SD, Diem S, et al. Efficacy of Vaginal Estradiol or Vaginal Moisturizer vs Placebo for Treating Postmenopausal Vulvovaginal Symptoms: A Randomized Clinical Trial. JAMA Intern Med 2018;178(5):681–90.
107. Lethaby A, Ayeleke RO, Roberts H. Local oestrogen for vaginal atrophy in postmenopausal women. Cochrane Database Syst Rev 2016;2016(8):CD001500.
108. Diem SJ, Guthrie KA, Mitchell CM, et al. Effects of vaginal estradiol tablets and moisturizer on menopause-specific quality of life and mood in healthy postmenopausal women with vaginal symptoms: a randomized clinical trial. Menopause 2018;25(10):1086–93.
109. Weisberg E, Ayton R, Darling G, et al. Endometrial and vaginal effects of low-dose estradiol delivered by vaginal ring or vaginal tablet. Climacteric 2005; 8(1):83–92.
110. Notelovitz M, Funk S, Nanavati N, et al. Estradiol absorption from vaginal tablets in postmenopausal women. Obstet Gynecol 2002;99(4):556–62.
111. Rioux JE, Devlin C, Gelfand MM, et al. 17beta-estradiol vaginal tablet versus conjugated equine estrogen vaginal cream to relieve menopausal atrophic vaginitis. Menopause 2000;7(3):156–61.
112. Simon J, Nachtigall L, Ulrich LG, et al. Endometrial safety of ultra-low-dose estradiol vaginal tablets. Obstet Gynecol 2010;116(4):876–83.
113. Naessen T, Rodriguez-Macias K. Endometrial thickness and uterine diameter not affected by ultralow doses of 17beta-estradiol in elderly women. Am J Obstet Gynecol 2002;186(5):944–7.
114. Crandall CJ, Hovey KM, Andrews CA, et al. Breast cancer, endometrial cancer, and cardiovascular events in participants who used vaginal estrogen in the Women's Health Initiative Observational Study. Menopause 2018;25(1):11–20.
115. Biehl C, Plotsker O, Mirkin S. A systematic review of the efficacy and safety of vaginal estrogen products for the treatment of genitourinary syndrome of menopause. Menopause 2019;26(4):431–53.
116. Vinogradova Y, Coupland C, Hippisley-Cox J. Use of hormone replacement therapy and risk of venous thromboembolism: nested case-control studies using the QResearch and CPRD databases. BMJ 2019;364:k4810.
117. Guthrie JR, Dennerstein L, Taffe JR, et al. The menopausal transition: a 9-year prospective population-based study. The Melbourne Women's Midlife Health Project. Climacteric 2004;7(4):375–89.
118. Lee JS, Ettinger B, Stanczyk FZ, et al. Comparison of methods to measure low serum estradiol levels in postmenopausal women. J Clin Endocrinol Metab 2006;91(10):3791–7.
119. Santen RJ, Pinkerton JV, Conaway M, et al. Treatment of urogenital atrophy with low-dose estradiol: preliminary results. Menopause 2002;9(3):179–87.
120. Mandel FP, Geola FL, Meldrum DR, et al. Biological effects of various doses of vaginally administered conjugated equine estrogens in postmenopausal women. J Clin Endocrinol Metab 1983;57(1):133–9.
121. Rigg LA, Hermann H, Yen SS. Absorption of estrogens from vaginal creams. N Engl J Med 1978;298(4):195–7.
122. The 2020 genitourinary syndrome of menopause position statement of The North American Menopause Society. Menopause 2020;27(9):976–92.
123. Bachmann GA, Komi JO, Ospemifene Study G. Ospemifene effectively treats vulvovaginal atrophy in postmenopausal women: results from a pivotal phase 3 study. Menopause 2010;17(3):480–6.

124. Portman DJ, Bachmann GA, Simon JA, et al. Ospemifene, a novel selective estrogen receptor modulator for treating dyspareunia associated with postmenopausal vulvar and vaginal atrophy. Menopause 2013;20(6):623–30.
125. Constantine G, Graham S, Portman DJ, et al. Female sexual function improved with ospemifene in postmenopausal women with vulvar and vaginal atrophy: results of a randomized, placebo-controlled trial. Climacteric 2015;18(2):226–32.
126. Goldstein I, Simon JA, Kaunitz AM, et al. Effects of ospemifene on genitourinary health assessed by prospective vulvar-vestibular photography and vaginal/vulvar health indices. Menopause 2019;26(9):994–1001.
127. Simon JA, Lin VH, Radovich C, et al. One-year long-term safety extension study of ospemifene for the treatment of vulvar and vaginal atrophy in postmenopausal women with a uterus. Menopause 2013;20(4):418–27.
128. Martel C, Labrie F, Archer DF, et al. Serum steroid concentrations remain within normal postmenopausal values in women receiving daily 6.5mg intravaginal prasterone for 12 weeks. J Steroid Biochem Mol Biol 2016;159:142–53.
129. Labrie F, Derogatis L, Archer DF, et al. Effect of Intravaginal Prasterone on Sexual Dysfunction in Postmenopausal Women with Vulvovaginal Atrophy. J Sex Med 2015;12(12):2401–12.
130. Labrie F, Archer DF, Koltun W, et al. Efficacy of intravaginal dehydroepiandrosterone (DHEA) on moderate to severe dyspareunia and vaginal dryness, symptoms of vulvovaginal atrophy, and of the genitourinary syndrome of menopause. Menopause 2018;25(11):1339–53.
131. Rymer J, Chapman MG, Fogelman I, et al. A study of the effect of tibolone on the vagina in postmenopausal women. Maturitas 1994;18(2):127–33.
132. Salvatore S, Leone R, Maggiore U, Athanasiou S, et al. Histological study on the effects of microablative fractional CO2 laser on atrophic vaginal tissue: an ex vivo study. Menopause 2015;22(8):845–9.
133. Li FG, Maheux-Lacroix S, Deans R, et al. Effect of Fractional Carbon Dioxide Laser vs Sham Treatment on Symptom Severity in Women With Postmenopausal Vaginal Symptoms: A Randomized Clinical Trial. JAMA 2021;326(14):1381–9.
134. Paraiso MFR, Ferrando CA, Sokol ER, et al. A randomized clinical trial comparing vaginal laser therapy to vaginal estrogen therapy in women with genitourinary syndrome of menopause: The VeLVET Trial. Menopause 2020;27(1):50–6.
135. Cruz VL, Steiner ML, Pompei LM, et al. Randomized, double-blind, placebo-controlled clinical trial for evaluating the efficacy of fractional CO2 laser compared with topical estriol in the treatment of vaginal atrophy in postmenopausal women. Menopause 2018;25(1):21–8.
136. Alshiek J, Garcia B, Minassian V, et al. Vaginal Energy-Based Devices. Female Pelvic Med Reconstr Surg 2020;26(5):287–98.
137. ACOG. Fractional Laser Treatment of Vulvovaginal Atrophy and U.S.Food and Drug Administration Clearance. 2018. Available at: https://www.acog.org/clinical-information/policy-and-position-statements/position-statements/2018/fractional-laser-treatment-of-vulvovaginal-atrophy-and-us-food-and-drug-administration-clearance. Accessed May 2021.
138. Kravitz HM, Ganz PA, Bromberger J, et al. Sleep difficulty in women at midlife: a community survey of sleep and the menopausal transition. Menopause 2003;10(1):19–28.
139. Kravitz HM, Joffe H. Sleep during the perimenopause: a SWAN story. Obstet Gynecol Clin North Am 2011;38(3):567–86.

140. Baker FC, de Zambotti M, Colrain IM, et al. Sleep problems during the menopausal transition: prevalence, impact, and management challenges. Nat Sci Sleep 2018;10:73–95.
141. Gava G, Orsili I, Alvisi S, et al. Cognition, Mood and Sleep in Menopausal Transition: The Role of Menopause Hormone Therapy. Medicina (Kaunas) 2019; 55(10):668.
142. Cintron D, Lipford M, Larrea-Mantilla L, et al. Efficacy of menopausal hormone therapy on sleep quality: systematic review and meta-analysis. Endocrine 2017;55(3):702–11.
143. Pinkerton JV, Pan K, Abraham L, et al. Sleep parameters and health-related quality of life with bazedoxifene/conjugated estrogens: a randomized trial. Menopause 2014;21(3):252–9.
144. Yurcheshen ME, Guttuso T Jr, McDermott M, et al. Effects of gabapentin on sleep in menopausal women with hot flashes as measured by a Pittsburgh Sleep Quality Index factor scoring model. J Womens Health (Larchmt) 2009;18(9): 1355–60.
145. Freeman EW, Sammel MD, Lin H, et al. Associations of hormones and menopausal status with depressed mood in women with no history of depression. Arch Gen Psychiatry 2006;63(4):375–82.
146. Schmidt PJ, Haq N, Rubinow DR. A longitudinal evaluation of the relationship between reproductive status and mood in perimenopausal women. Am J Psychiatry 2004;161(12):2238–44.
147. Hickey M, Schoenaker DA, Joffe H, et al. Depressive symptoms across the menopause transition: findings from a large population-based cohort study. Menopause 2016;23(12):1287–93.
148. Maki PM, Kornstein SG, Joffe H, et al. Guidelines for the Evaluation and Treatment of Perimenopausal Depression: Summary and Recommendations. J Womens Health (Larchmt) 2019;28(2):117–34.
149. Maki PM, Kornstein SG, Joffe H, et al. Guidelines for the evaluation and treatment of perimenopausal depression: summary and recommendations. Menopause 2018;25(10):1069–85.
150. Clayton AH, Kornstein SG, Dunlop BW, et al. Efficacy and safety of desvenlafaxine 50 mg/d in a randomized, placebo-controlled study of perimenopausal and postmenopausal women with major depressive disorder. J Clin Psychiatry 2013; 74(10):1010–7.
151. Kornstein SG, Jiang Q, Reddy S, et al. Short-term efficacy and safety of desvenlafaxine in a randomized, placebo-controlled study of perimenopausal and postmenopausal women with major depressive disorder. J Clin Psychiatry 2010; 71(8):1088–96.
152. Willi J, Ehlert U. Assessment of perimenopausal depression: A review. J Affect Disord 2019;249:216–22.
153. Crandall CJ, Manson JE, Hohensee C, et al. Association of genetic variation in the tachykinin receptor 3 locus with hot flashes and night sweats in the Women's Health Initiative Study. Menopause 2017;24(3):252–61.
154. Jayasena CN, Comninos AN, Stefanopoulou E, et al. Neurokinin B administration induces hot flushes in women. Sci Rep 2015;5:8466.
155. Skorupskaite K, George JT, Veldhuis JD, et al. Neurokinin 3 Receptor Antagonism Reveals Roles for Neurokinin B in the Regulation of Gonadotropin Secretion and Hot Flashes in Postmenopausal Women. Neuroendocrinology 2018; 106(2):148–57.

156. Prague JK, Roberts RE, Comninos AN, et al. Neurokinin 3 receptor antagonism as a novel treatment for menopausal hot flushes: a phase 2, randomised, double-blind, placebo-controlled trial. Lancet 2017;389(10081):1809–20.
157. Fraser GL, Lederman S, Waldbaum A, et al. A phase 2b, randomized, placebo-controlled, double-blind, dose-ranging study of the neurokinin 3 receptor antagonist fezolinetant for vasomotor symptoms associated with menopause. Menopause 2020;27(4):382–92.
158. Depypere H, Timmerman D, Donders G, et al. Treatment of Menopausal Vasomotor Symptoms With Fezolinetant, a Neurokinin 3 Receptor Antagonist: A Phase 2a Trial. J Clin Endocrinol Metab 2019;104(12):5893–905.
159. Santoro N, Waldbaum A, Lederman S, et al. Effect of the neurokinin 3 receptor antagonist fezolinetant on patient-reported outcomes in postmenopausal women with vasomotor symptoms: results of a randomized, placebo-controlled, double-blind, dose-ranging study (VESTA). Menopause 2020;27(12):1350–6.
160. Lensen S, Archer D, Bell RJ, et al. A core outcome set for vasomotor symptoms associated with menopause: the COMMA (Core Outcomes in Menopause) global initiative. Menopause 2021;28(8):852–8.
161. Lensen S, Bell RJ, Carpenter JS, et al. A core outcome set for genitourinary symptoms associated with menopause: the COMMA (Core Outcomes in Menopause) global initiative. Menopause 2021;28(8):859–66.

Quality of Life in Primary Hyperparathyroidism

Cristiana Cipriani, MD, PhD[a,*], Luisella Cianferotti, MD, PhD[b]

KEYWORDS

• Quality of life • Primary hyperparathyroidism • Neuropsychiatric • Neurologic
• Cognition

KEY POINTS

- Impairment in quality of life is extensively reported in patients with primary hyperparathyroidism.
- Specific questionnaires may be used to assess quality of life, as well as to screen for neuropsychiatric and cognitive manifestations.
- Physical and functional domains of the quality of life, as well as the general health perception are reduced in primary hyperparathyroidism.
- Prospective studies and randomized controlled trials (RCTs) did not show consistent results on the improvement of neuropsychiatric symptoms and cognitive dysfunction after surgery.
- Quality of life overall increased after surgery in RCTs but results are heterogeneous.

INTRODUCTION

Primary hyperparathyroidism (PHPT) is one of the most common endocrine disorders. Clinical hallmarks of the disease include the presence of hypercalcemia and elevated or inappropriately normal serum parathyroid hormone (PTH) levels. Complications in target organs, such as chronic kidney disease, kidney stones, osteoporosis, and fragility fractures, are classically and commonly observed, even in the absence of symptoms. Noteworthy, other organs may be involved. Indeed, calcium receptors (ie, calcium sensing receptor) and PTH receptors (PTHR1 and PTHR2) are widely expressed throughout multiple organs and tissues, so that high calcium and PTH levels per se could directly modulate numerous physiologic functions.[1]

As learned by clinical experience, severe PHPT may present as a life-threatening condition comprising cardiovascular, neurologic, neuromuscular, and psychiatric

[a] Department of Clinical, Internal, Anesthesiological and Cardiovascular Sciences, Sapienza University of Rome, Viale del Policlinico 155, Rome 00161, Italy; [b] Department of Experimental and Clinical Biomedical Sciences "Mario Serio", University of Florence, Viale GB Morgagni 50, Florence 50134, Italy
* Corresponding author.
E-mail address: cristiana.cipriani@gmail.com

Endocrinol Metab Clin N Am 51 (2022) 837–852
https://doi.org/10.1016/j.ecl.2022.04.007

issues.[2] Patients may complain of depression, anxiety, sleep disturbances, and altered mental function or may present with delirium and/or psychosis.[1] Additionally, substantial data in recent decades has shown that complications involving the neuropsychiatric and cognitive system, may be commonly observed in the 3 phenotypes of PHPT, namely the symptomatic, asymptomatic, and normocalcemic.[3] Eventually, quality of life (QoL) is impaired.[4]

The administration of generic or disease-specific questionnaires in clinical studies have demonstrated neurobehavioral issues and cognitive impairment in PHPT patients even in the absence of overt neuropsychiatric disease.[4] Data have shown that patients with mild PHPT are at higher risk of presenting with symptoms of depression and anxiety compared with healthy age and sex-matched subjects.[1,5–7] Cognitive function, including memory, attention, concentration, and executive functions, may be impaired, frequently in association with depressive and anxiety symptoms.[1,3,8] Several domains of QoL, including physical capacity, vitality, social, and emotional functions, are reduced in PHPT.[1,4] These results have been observed in both mild and normocalcemic PHPT, with possible different presentation between the 2 phenotypes.[4,9–11]

Factors considered as potentially influencing neuropsychiatric complications and QoL in PHPT were age, comorbidities, serum calcium, and PTH levels but no conclusive results were reported.[1] Finally, parathyroidectomy (PTX) was associated with a better outcome compared with clinical observation in terms of QoL in some but not all RCTs.[12–15]

Evaluation

Several tools have been used in clinical studies to assess neuropsychiatric symptoms, cognition, and QoL in PHPT.[3,4,16,17] Questionnaires investigating the presence and severity of depressive symptoms, state and trait anxiety, and the global assessment of the psychological distress associated with depression, anxiety, and somatization were used.[12,18–20] One of the most frequently used depression questionnaire is the Patient Health Questionnaire-9 (PHQ-9).[5,20] This is based on the 9 criteria used for the diagnosis of depression derived from the Diagnostic and Statistical Manual of Mental Disorders IV, with each of one being scored by frequency.

Additionally, testing has focused on other psychological dimensions, such as obsessive-compulsive disorder, suicidal ideation, interpersonal sensitivity, phobia, hostility, paranoid ideation, and psychoticism.[6,12–14]

Cognition has been investigated by questionnaires assessing memory as immediate and delayed recall word list memory, spatial working memory and error monitoring, and visual memory.[4,18,19] Intellectual quotient, nonverbal abstraction, visual concentration and attention, auditory attention, processing speed and mental manipulation were assessed by specific questionnaires, as well.[4,18,19,21]

Clinical studies on QoL in PHPT have used 2 main instruments, the parathyroidectomy assessment of symptoms (PAS) score and the Short Form Health Surveys (SF-36; **Table 1**). More recently, the health-related QoL questionnaire for PHPT patients (PHPQoL-16), and the 15-D instrument were used[4,16,17,22] (see **Table 1**).

In the 1990s to early 2000s, Pasieka and colleagues validated a disease-specific questionnaire assessing nonspecific symptoms of PHPT, such as bone and joint pain, muscle function, memory, and other neuropsychiatric symptoms.[22] The PAS score was calculated by a questionnaire assessing the presence and degree of severity (on a visual analog scale) of 13 symptoms (see **Table 1**).[22]

The SF-36 is the most commonly used questionnaire to assess health perception and health-related QoL in PHPT. The validated short-form (SF-12) was used in one

Table 1
Clinical tools for assessing quality of life in PHPT

Tool	Disease-specific PAS	PHPQoL-16	Non-disease specific SF-36	15D instrument
Characteristics	• 13 items assessing vague and non-specific symptoms of PHPT (pain, memory issues, neuropsychiatric symptoms, itchy) • Symptoms are evaluated at the time the patient responds on a VAS scale (0-100)	• 16 items • 2 domains Physical Emotional • Good association with SF-36 and the PWBI scores	• 35 items • 8 health dimensions Physical: Physical Functioning, Role Physical, Bodily Pain, General Health Physical component summary (PCS) Mental: Vitality, Social Functioning, Role Emotional, Mental Health Mental component summary (MCS) • Assessment of change in health over time	• 15 dimensions mobility, vision, hearing, breathing, sleeping, eating, speech, excretion, usual activities, mental function, discomfort and symptoms, depression, distress, vitality, sexual activity
Advantages	• Ease of administration • Well validated • Disease-specific	• Ease of administration • Short questions and few response categories • Disease-specific	• Ease of administration • Widely validated • Translated in many languages • Employed in many endocrine disorders	• Ease of administration • Well validated • Employed in many endocrine disorders
Limits	• Lack of longitudinal data from RCTs	• Few data • Lack of long-term longitudinal data in PHPT	• Not disease-specific	• Few data in PHPT • Not disease-specific • Lack of long-term longitudinal data in PHPT

Abbreviations: PAS, parathyroid assessment of symptoms; PHPQoL-16, health-related quality of life questionnaire for PHPT patients; PWBI, Psychological Well-Being Index; SF-36, Short Form Health Surveys study, as well.[23] Since its validation, the SF-36 has been widely used in the last 3 decades because of its reliability and ease of use.[24] Additionally, it has been translated in several languages and used in different populations and in many endocrine disorders.[25,26] The questionnaire is composed of 35 items exploring physical and mental dimensions of health, and the general health (see **Table 1**).[27]

Interestingly, Mihai and colleagues demonstrated a good correlation between PAS score and the physical and mental component scores of the SF-36 in a prospective case-series study in 101 patients with PHPT in United Kingdom.[28]

The PHPQoL-16 was recently developed as a tool for specifically evaluating QoL in PHPT.[16,29] It is a 16-item questionnaire exploring 2 main domains, namely the physical and the emotional domain.[29] Webb and colleagues reported a moderate-to-high association among PHPQoL scores and SF-36 and the Psychological Well-Being Index scores, as well as the personal health status perception in a study involving 182 patients with PHPT[16] (see **Table 1**).

The 15D instrument is 15-dimension questionnaire assessing 5 levels of neuropsychological, cognitive and physical symptoms and functions.[30] Its use in PHPT was evaluated by Ryhänen and colleagues in a prospective intervention study involving 124 patients.[17] Authors showed significant impairment in the QoL and amelioration after surgery in PHPT patients but no comparison with other instruments for the evaluation of QoL was performed.[17]

Current Evidence

Neuropsychiatric and cognitive symptoms in primary hyperparathyroidism

Clinical studies have demonstrated that neuropsychiatric disease and symptoms are more prevalent in PHPT patients compared with controls.[13] Depression, anxiety, psychosis, personality changes, fatigue, impaired vitality, altered social and emotional functions, and sleep disturbances are the most commonly reported.[4] Unfortunately, there is heterogeneity among studies in the tools used to assess neuropsychiatric symptoms, and the populations studied in terms inclusion/exclusion criteria, particularly as far as phenotype of PHPT, age range, concomitant neuropsychiatric disorders and/or disease possibly influencing the neuropsychiatric system. Hence, data from clinical studies describe a prevalence of depression and/or depressive symptoms ranging from 20% to 62%.[5,6,9,10,19,31–33] Anxiety is reported in 20% to 53% of patients with PHPT.[6,8,10,19,31,32] In normocalcemic PHPT, a corresponding figure of 38% for depression and 61% for anxiety is described by one prospective study.[10]

As far as cognition, the most prevalent symptoms in patients with PHPT are impaired memory, attention, verbal fluency and executive function, dementia, loss of initiative and concentration.[3] Significant impairment in cognition was observed in 24% to 47% of patients with PHPT in clinical studies.[10,29,31,32] A study by Bannani and colleagues reported a 28% prevalence of memory loss in normocalcemic PHPT patients.[10]

Studies have shown discordant results based on geography in terms of the prevalence of neuropsychiatric symptoms and impairment in cognition as clinical manifestations of PHPT. A recent observational study by Liu and colleagues in a US cohort reported no cases of overt depression, as assessed by the Centers for Epidemiologic Studies Depression Scale, nor impaired cognition among 36 postmenopausal women with mild hypercalcemic ($n = 29$) and normocalcemic ($n = 7$) PHPT.[34] Additionally, the PHPT group did not score significantly different in terms of depressive symptoms compared with age and sex-matched subjects with thyroid disease.[34] These data were in line with those previously observed by the same group in a case-control study involving 39 postmenopausal women with PHPT.[18] In this study, the assessment of depression, state and trait anxiety revealed higher values compared with 89 postmenopausal controls but no clinical diagnosis of depression and/or anxiety was made.[18] Verbal memory and nonverbal abstraction were altered in PHPT compared with healthy subjects, whereas others such as visual memory, concentration, auditory attention, and mental manipulation were not.[18] In another US cohort of 212 women and men with PHPT, Roman and colleagues described no baseline cognitive impairment compared with the control group, whereas the depression and anxiety scores were mildly elevated.[19]

Conversely, Yadav and colleagues observed a high proportion of patients with neuropsychiatric symptoms in 3 Indian cohorts of PHPT patients assessed from 1990 to 2016, with prevalence ranging from 10.7% to 29.4%.[35] Similar data were observed by Prasarttong-Osoth and colleagues in a cohort of PHPT patients from Thailand; 8.9% presented with altered consciousness and 2.2% with psychosis.[36] Finally, Eufrazino and colleagues reported a 22% prevalence of depression in a Brazilian cohort of 27 otherwise asymptomatic PHPT subjects.[33]

Hence, geographic differences in the rate of neuropsychiatric symptoms in PHPT could be ascribed to the well-known relative prevalence of the 3 phenotypes of the disease, namely the symptomatic, asymptomatic, and normocalcemic, throughout the world.[37,38] This point has been directly associated with diverse clinical approaches to general medicine and, specifically, to metabolic bone disease among countries.[37]

Quality of life in primary hyperparathyroidism

QoL was assessed in many observational and intervention studies in the last 4 decades.[4] Additionally, 4 RCTs on the effect of PTX versus observation in PHPT have been published, with assessments of QoL among the primary endpoints.[12–15] Of these RCTs, 2 reported baseline data on QoL in PHPT versus non-PHPT subjects.[12,13] **Table 2** summarizes data from the RCTs and the most recent (10 years) observational studies.

Baseline data on QoL from RCTs showed heterogeneous results. However, this point may be associated with the lack of a control group in the RCTs, and the choice of comparing baseline results in PHPT with normative data from the general population. Bollerslev and colleagues compared baseline results from the SF-36 questionnaire in PHPT patients with data from the Swedish population.[13] The authors reported significantly lower scores in PHPT in 4 psychological domains, namely vitality, social functioning, role emotional, and mental health compared with the general population.[13] Hence, the mental component summary (MCS) score was significantly lower in PHPT (46.3 ± 12.4) versus the reference Swedish population (51.0 ± 10.4)[13]. Differently, Rao and colleagues did not specifically compare SF-36 values in the PHPT group with a reference population but rather stated that results were not different from those published elsewhere in patients without PHPT.[12]

Several observational (prospective and cross-sectional) studies have been published in the last decade and assessed QoL in PHPT patients in comparison with control cohorts of healthy subjects and/or the general or country-specific population (**Table 2**).[6,7,11,17,39,40] Collectively, these studies are concordant in showing a significant impairment in the psychological domains of QoL in patients with PHPT. Additionally, the detrimental effect of PHPT on the dimensions of QoL exploring the physical well-being were reported in almost all the studies.

A randomized double-blind study on the effect of vitamin D on QoL in patients who have undergone successful PTX compared baseline data in 135 PHPT patients with those from a cohort of 459 age-matched and sex-matched subjects from the Swedish SF-36 normative database.[40] The authors observed significantly lower values in all the

Table 2
Baseline data on quality of life in primary hyperparathyroidism from RCTs and the most recent (10-y) observational studies.

Study	Design	Patients	Age, yrs	Assessment	Baseline data
Rao et al,[12] 2004	RCT	53 F/M 42/11	range 50–75	SF-36	Scores in PHPT were similar to those of patients without PHPT
Bollerslev et al,[13] 2007	RCT	191 F/M 165/26	mean 64.2 ± 7.2	SF-36	Lower scores in 4 mental domains and in MCS in PHPT vs controls
Weber et al,[6] 2013	Prospective intervention	194 F/M 153/41	mean 58.5 ± 14.4	SF-36	Lower PCS and MCS scores in PHPT vs controls and vs the healthy German population
Rolighed et al,[43] 2014	Cross-sectional	58 F/M 47/11	range 55–62	SF-36	Lower scores in all 8 domains of the SF-36, MCS and PCS in PHPT vs controls
Ryhanen et al,[17] 2015	Prospective intervention	124 F/M 101/23	mean 65 ± 10.2	15-D	Lower score in PHPT vs general population in 13 dimensions; mental function, discomfort and symptoms, depression, distress, vitality, excretion, usual and sexual activities were severely affected
Aberg et al,[44] 2015	Randomized double-blind study	135 F/M 109/36	range 30–50	SF-36	Lower score in all 8 domains of the SF-36, MCS and PCS in PHPT vs reference country-specific population
Yilmaz et al,[7] 2017	Case-control	37 F/M 30/7	mean 53.9 ± 7.3	SF-36	Lower score in PHPT vs controls in physical functioning, mental health, social functioning, emotional role
Voss et al,[11] 2020	Case-control	20 postmenopausal women 7 hypercalcemic PHPT 13 NPHPT	mean 63 ± 13	SF-36	Lower scores in metal health domain in hypercalcemic PHPT vs controls; lower scores in the general health in NPHPT vs controls

Abbreviations: SF-36, Short Form Health Survey; MCS, Mental Component Summary; PCS, Physical Component Summary; WHO-5, World Health Organisation Five Well-Being Index survey; PHPQoL, Primary Hyperparathyroidism Quality of Life; NPHPT, normocalcemic PHPT.

8 domains of the SF-36 questionnaire, and consequently in the MCS and the Physical Component Summary in PHPT subjects versus the reference population.[40] Similar results were reported in the studies by Weber and colleagues and Rolighed and colleagues performed in a German and a Danish cohort, respectively.[6,39] Weber and colleagues studied 194 PHPT patients in which QoL, assessed by the SF-36, was significantly reduced in all the domains compared with a control age-matched and sex-matched group and a country-specific reference cohort.[6] Rolighed and colleagues compared the SF-36 data of a cohort 58 PHPT patients with a group of 58 control subjects recruited from the same population.[39] The authors found an overall reduction in all the SF-36 scores, as well as a lower well-being and higher prevalence of depression, assessed by the World Health Organisation Five Well-Being Index survey in PHPT versus controls.[39]

Interestingly, the most recent literature shows an overall global agreement in defining the impairment in QoL in PHPT patients. In accordance with studies from the United States, United Kingdom, and Northern Europe, recent studies from Turkey and Brazil showed reductions in QoL in PHPT.[7,11] Yilmaz and colleagues observed significant reductions in the physical functioning, mental health, social functioning, and emotional role in a Turkish cohort of 37 young adults with PHPT.[7] Voss and colleagues reported SF-36 data from a Brazilian cohort of 20 subjects with both hypercalcemic and normocalcemic PHPT; the mental health domain and the general health perception were affected in the 2 groups, respectively.[11]

The overall data demonstrate that QoL is significantly impaired in PHPT. The use of different instruments and the assessment of patients of both sexes and different age groups have invariably confirmed these results. In contrast to other manifestations and complications of the disease, no geographic trend in the impairment in QoL seems to be evident from clinical studies.

Effect of Surgery on Quality of Life

PTX is the primary treatment of symptomatic PHPT with classic signs and symptoms (ie, bone and kidney involvement). Criteria elaborated by an international panel of experts have been developed since 1990 and revised on a regular basis to select asymptomatic patients with mild disease who may benefit the most by removal of affected gland/glands.[41,42,43] Neuromuscular and neuropsychiatric symptoms, accounted within the nontraditional manifestations of the disease, along with physical and work performance and QoL, have not been included in these guidelines, so far, because of the lack of adequate evidence.[41,42,43] Indeed, although many observational studies, mainly monocentric and retrospective, generally demonstrated a beneficial effect of PTX on the nonspecific symptoms in patients with complicated/more severe PHPT, few RCTs, mostly with a short-term and medium-term assessment, have been carried out on the effect of PTX on QoL in mild disease.

Evidence from observational studies

Observational studies, which have included mainly patients who met the recommendations for surgery, that is, patients with severe disease (ie, with moderate-severe hypercalcemia, osteoporosis with or without fragility fractures, kidney disease), demonstrated an overall beneficial effect of surgery on several aspects of QoL, psychological function, and cognitive improvement.

Since the first observations of the improvement in neurocognitive alterations in PHPT after surgery,[44] in the last 2 decades, many observational studies, both retrospective and prospective, and mostly including patients with symptomatic/complicated PHPT, have repeatedly shown a beneficial effect of PTX in terms of nonspecific/QoL-related symptoms. These studies have been included in several meta-analyses focusing on QoL outcomes in PHPT after successful surgical treatment.

A meta-analysis published in 2015 included only 6 prospective studies systematically assessing QoL by SF-36 and/or Pasieka scores in patients with PHPT before and up to 6 months/1 year after successful PTX.[28,45–50] All SF-36 derived scores (vitality, physical functioning, bodily pain, general health, role physical, role emotional, role social, and mental health) were assessed in 238 patients,[46,48–50] as well as the Pasieka scores (feeling tired, feeling thirsty, mood swings, joint pains, irritability, feeling blues, feeling weak, itchy, forgetful, headache, abdominal pain, bone pain, ability to move off chair) assessed in 203 patients[28,47,50] improved significantly after surgery ($P < 0.001$ vs baseline for each item). These findings let the authors conclude that surgical treatment significantly ameliorated QoL in patients with PHPT in the short-medium term.[45]

When a depression-specific questionnaire was used (ie, the PHQ-9), scores showed improvement both in somatic and cognitive domains after surgery in patients with PHPT.[5,20] Even sleep quality, which is compromised in untreated PHPT, improved in the short term after surgery.[51] Walker and colleagues demonstrated an improvement of compromised neurocognitive features, in particular affecting verbal memory and nonverbal abstraction, in mild PHPT after surgery, as assessed by a comprehensive test battery.[18]

Long-term PAS assessment demonstrated that the benefits, at least in part, persisted over time (ie, 3 and 10 years after surgery).[52,53]

A multicenter longitudinal study examined QoL-related outcomes within the Swiss PHPT Cohort Study, which enrolled 332 consecutive patients with PHPT in several referral centers. The authors demonstrated that the elevated depression and anxiety scores and cognitive dysfunction, which are often associated, may be mitigated by PTX, which was performed in 153 (46%) who met surgical criteria.[32] Other multicenter studies had previously shown similar results,[6] even in surgically treated mild[54,55] or in normocalcemic PHPT.[10]

The type of surgery (robotic-assisted PTX vs minimally invasive PTX) does not seem to influence the outcome of surgery in terms of QoL,[56] as well as vitamin D supplementation.[40]

All in all, these studies indicate that patients with moderate-to-severe forms of PHPT and/or complicated disease are likely to show nonspecific symptomatic benefit from surgical treatment. The evidence is more limited for mild PHPT without the classic bone and kidney involvement.

Evidence from RCTs

Since 2004, 6 trials have been carried out in "asymptomatic" patients with PHPT who did not meet correspondent consensus conference criteria for undergoing PTX, as summarized in **Table 3**. All of these studies enrolled subjects older than 50 years, and predominantly postmenopausal women, according to the epidemiology of PHPT. SF-36 was overall the most used test for QoL assessment across these studies. The first study by Rao and colleagues included 53 apparently "healthy" patients with mild disease randomly assigned to either PTX or routine monitoring, according to National Institute of Health guidelines, followed-up to 24 months. Although a significant deterioration in 5 out of 9 SF-36 derived QoL-related domains (ie, energy, social functioning, physical and emotional problem, and overall health perception) was demonstrated in the patients who were followed without surgery, just one domain (physical function) was compromised in patients cured by PTX.[12] A modest yet significant

Table 3
Randomized controlled trials in patients with mild/asymptomatic primary hyperparathyroidism assessing the effect of parathyroidectomy on quality of life, neurologic and physical function versus conservative management

Author and year of Publication	Sample size (N of Enrolled patients at baseline)	Women/ Men Ratio	Follow-up (N of patients at Follow-up)	Assessment Tools	Results
Rao et al,[12] 2004	53	42/11	2 y (N = 53)	SF-36, SCL-90R	PTXG vs OG: significant improvement in emotional role function, social function, anxiety and phobia OG: significant deterioration in physical problem, emotional problem, social functioning, energy and health perception
Bollerslev et al,[13] 2007	191	165/16	2 y (N = 99)	SF-36, CPRS	PTXG: significant improvement in mental health score at 1 y but not at 2 y OG: significant improvement in mental health score at 2 y PTXG: significant improvement only in role emotional
Ambrogini et al,[14] 2007	50	46/4	1 y (N = 50)	SF-36, SCL-90R	PTXG vs OG: significant improvement in general health, bodily pain, vitality, mental health
Perrier et al,[60] 2009	18	15/3	6 mo (N = 18)	fMRI, sleep assessment (actigraphy and questionnaires), neuropsychological test battery	PTXG: significant improvement in sleep and decrease in sleepiness associated with executive function
Morris et al,[61] 2010	18	15/3	6 mo (N = 18)	6-min walk test, 50-foot walk test, repeated sit-to-stand test	PTXG: significant improvement in the 6-min walk test
Pretorius et al,[15] 2021	191	165/16	10 y (N = 129)	SF-36, CPRS	PTXG vs OG: significant improvement in vitality but not in the psychological domains in the long-term Psychological function improved both in the PTXG and OG in the long-term, with no differences between the 2 groups Improvement in QoL observed in PTXG at 1 y waned over time

Abbreviations: PTX-G, PTX group; OG, observation group; SF-36, 36-item Short Form health survey; SCL-90R, Symptom Check List-90-Revised; CPRS, Comprehensive Psychopathological Rating Scale; fMRI, functional Magnetic Resonance Imaging.

improvement in QoL and psychological function was observed after PTX in mild PHPT. Although a possible placebo effect of surgery could not be excluded, these findings demonstrated that in the long-term PTX could provide some benefit in QoL in asymptomatic patients.[12] A following RCT in a similar magnitude of patients with asymptomatic PHPT demonstrated a beneficial effect of PTX on QoL at just 1 year of follow-up.[14] In particular, bodily pain, vitality, mental health, and general health improved in treated patients as compared to untreated ones.[14] Conversely, in the same year, a multicenter trial including patients from Denmark, Sweden and Norway (Scandinavian Study on PHPT, SIPH) which randomized a larger cohort of patients, failed to show any improvement in QoL after PTX in patients with mild disease when compared to the medical observation group, as assessed by SF-36 and the psychopathological Rating Scale (CPRS).[13] Nonetheless, a slight but significant decrease in the SF-36 physical domains was shown in the untreated group in the 2-year time of observation, while no change was noticed in the operation group.[13] Although treated patients had a slight improvement in mental health scores at 1 but not at 2 years of observation, the delta over time in the domain role emotional were higher with respect to the medical observation group.[13] Smaller RCTs have subsequently assessed QoL by means of additional tests. In the study by Perrier and colleagues, a small group of patients with mild PHPT enrolled in a referral endocrine surgery center were randomized to conservative management or PTX and evaluated by functional magnetic resonance imaging and sleep assessment, along with a validated neuropsychological battery up to 6 months.[57] An improvement in sleep and decrease in sleepiness, which was associated with executive function, were demonstrated in subject cured by surgery.[57] The same groups were also analyzed for physical performance.[58] All patients were tested by means of 6-minute walk test, 50-foot walk test, and repeated sit-to-stand times. Although the 50-foot walk test and sit-to-stand tests remained unchanged, a significant improvement was observed in the 6-minute walk test in the treated group, just after 6 months after PTX, indicating that a recovery of physical function can be expected after surgery in mild disease.[58]

Nonetheless, a recent meta-analysis pooling the results of these RCTs failed to demonstrate an overall benefit on QoL-related parameters.[59]

These promising results were, in part, jeopardized by the finding that some observed benefits after PTX did not persist in the medium-term observation period (2 years). Moreover, earlier studies relied on generic questionnaires, nonspecific for the disease, whereas disease-specific questionnaires, such as PHPQoL, validated against PAS and made available only recently,[60] have still to be exploited in RCTs.

In 2021, the results of the multicenter SIPH study, with an observation period extended up to 10 years in 129 out of 191 enrolled subjects, were published.[15] After PTX, a significant although modest improvement in QoL was demonstrated in some domains, such as vitality but not in the psychological domains.[15] Indeed, psychological function as assessed by CPRS recovered both in the treated and untreated groups to a similar extent in the long-term, so that no differences were detected between them.[15] It is noteworthy that the improvement in QoL observed after 1 year, as in previous studies, was attenuated in the following years, demonstrating the need of long-term observation after an intervention, due to the bias of nonspecific benefits of surgery on general symptoms.[15,61] Besides these results, no deterioration in overall QoL was observed in the patients with untreated, persistent mild disease in the long-term, underlying the fact that, still, nonspecific symptoms cannot be included among the indications for surgery in mild PHPT.[15,61] Nonetheless, the fact that 50 patients (26% of the total randomized) were lost during the long-term follow up and 17 additional patients were crossed over to treatment, still remaining in the original analysis as "untreated" group for analyses due to the Intention-To-Treat principle, might have undermined the overall negative results. With this respect, the dropouts in the observation group could have had worse QoL as compared with treated individuals who were followed until the end of the study.[61] Moreover, the individuals who accepted randomization to PTX versus non-PTX could be different in terms of baseline systemic symptoms.

Although it is unlikely that large, long-term RCTs of this kind will be published in the near future, smaller trials using more disease-specific tests such as PHPQoL along with physical activity assessment are still needed in this field.

Effect of Cinacalcet on Quality of Life

Calcimimetic agents such as cinacalcet have been used in PHPT to effectively decrease moderate-to-severe hypercalcemia when surgical treatment is considered unfeasible. It has been clearly shown that, besides the control of hypercalcemia, no effect on overall disease (bone and kidney involvement) could be demonstrated.[62] To our knowledge, a systematic assessment of QoL was never included in the studies testing cinacalcet in PHPT. Only one recent clinical case report on the possible effect of cinacalcet on cognitive impairment in an elderly patient, as assessed by mini mental state examination has been published.[63] One observational study carried out in 110 Swedish patients with PHPT treated by PTX, has shown that the effective response to preoperative treatment with cinacalcet in terms of QoL-related parameters, cognitive function, and muscle strength might predict the effects of surgical normalization of hypercalcemia on systemic, nondisease-specific symptoms, especially in elderly patients.[64,65]

SUMMARY

Undeniably, patients with PHPT often present with various alterations of QoL and neuropsychiatric symptoms during active disease. It is difficult to dissect in humans whether nonspecific symptoms are due to hypercalcemia per se and/or high PTH levels, given the widespread presence of PTH receptors. These general manifestations, not classically related to mineral homeostasis, can be assessed by various tools. SF-36 has been the most used tool to test QoL in PHPT but also other questionnaires have been used in this regard, with some of them (PAS and PHPQoL) specifically designed and validated for the disease, which, unfortunately, have not been yet tested in RCTs. Interestingly, although a geographic trend seems evident as far as neurocognitive and psychiatric symptoms, with studies form the US reporting less severe involvement, there is an overall global agreement in reporting the reduction in QoL in PHPT.

Many longitudinal studies have demonstrated an overall general improvement in QoL after successful surgery. These studies mainly included patients with more severe forms of the disease, leading to the therapeutic choice of surgical treatment.

Meta-analyses have not examined subgroups of patients (ie, on the basis of age, sex, comorbidities) and failed to find cut-off values in order to recommend surgery based on the disease severity in terms of QoL. Some studies have shown that younger subjects are shown to benefit more from PTX in terms of QoL. This, indeed, has been suggested in some studies, such as the one by Caillard and colleagues, who found that patients younger than 70 and with a serum calcium more than 10.4 mg/dL display more pronounced improvement after surgery.[48] This may explain why some longitudinal studies and meta-analyses considering mild PHPT have failed to find significant benefits after surgery in QoL-related domains and neurocognitive symptoms.[66]

Moreover, patients dropouts in the long-term trials could have had differences in the symptoms at baseline hampering the results of the intention-to-treat analysis in the long term.[15]

Subanalyses in young versus elderly subjects and in women versus men are needed, as well as inclusion of other assessments, such as frailty in elders,[67] which could help to refine assessment of QoL in these subjects. In addition, studies of QoL with cinacalcet treatment, especially in elders, are needed, in order to assess whether just a modulation of serum calcium might modulate nonspecific symptoms and improve well-being in subjects not submitted to surgery.

Although it is unlikely that nonspecific symptoms will be included in recommendation for surgery in mild PHPT because of the lack of significant evidence available to date and the difficulty of obtaining additional results from large, long-term RCTs in the near future, it is advisable to systematically evaluate these symptoms in each patient with the aim to practice personalized medicine.

CLINICS CARE POINTS

- Neuropsychiatric symptoms, impaired cognition and quality of life (QoL) are common manifestations of primary hyperparathyroidism (PHPT).
- Numerous questionnaires have been used to assess these complications, with the 36-item Short Form health survey and the more disease-specific parathyroidectomy assessment of symptoms the most commonly used.
- Depression, anxiety, impaired memory, attention, concentration, and dementia are the symptoms most commonly reported.
- All mental domains of QoL may be impaired in PHPT; physical components of the QoL may be involved, as well.
- An overall general benefit of surgery on QoL was observed in observational studies.
- The psychological domains of QoL were usually improved after parathyroidectomy in RCTs in the mid-term; longer term (10-year) data demonstrated no difference between surgery and observation in the amelioration of QoL.
- Limited data on cinacalcet have demonstrated a possible positive effect of its preoperative use on QoL; long-term prospective studies are needed.
- The assessment of neuropsychiatric symptoms and QoL in PHPT patients is advisable in clinical practice.

DISCLOSURE

The authors have nothing to disclose.

REFERENCES

1. Chiodini I, Cairoli E, Palmieri S, et al. Non classical complications of primary hyperparathyroidism. Best Pract Res Clin Endocrinol Metab 2018;32(6):805–20.
2. Fitzpatrick LABJ. Acute primary hyperparathyroidism. Am J Med 1987;82(2) 275–82.
3. Lourida I, Thompson-Coon J, Dickens CM, et al. Parathyroid hormone, cognitive function and dementia: a systematic review. PLoS One 2015;10(5):e012757 [Electronic Resource].

4. Cipriani C, Romagnoli E, Cilli M, et al. Quality of life in patients with primary hyperparathyroidism. Expert Rev Pharmacoecon Outcomes Res 2014;14(1):113–21.
5. Kearns AE, Espiritu RP, Douglass KV, et al. Clinical characteristics and depression score response after parathyroidectomy in primary hyperparathyroidism. Clin Endocrinol 2019;91(3):464–70.
6. Weber TEJ, Messelhäuser U, Schiffmann L, et al. Parathyroidectomy, elevated depression scores, and suicidal ideation in patients with primary hyperparathyroidism: results of a prospective multicenter study. JAMA Surg 2013;148(2):109–15.
7. Yılmaz BA, Törüner FB, Değertekin CK, et al. Neuropsychological changes and health-related quality of life in patients with asymptomatic primary hyperparathyroidism. Asemptomatik primer hiperparatiroidizmi olan hastalarda nöropsiklojik değişiklikler ve yaşam kalitesi 2017;21(1):9–14.
8. Shah-Becker S, Derr J, Oberman BS, et al. Early neurocognitive improvements following parathyroidectomy for primary hyperparathyroidism. Laryngoscope 2018;128(3):775–80.
9. Veras A, Maia J, Mesquita P, et al. Lower quality of life in longstanding mild primary hyperparathyroidism. Arq Bras Endocrinol Metabol 2013;57(2):139–43.
10. Bannani SA-O, Christou N, Guérin C, et al. Effect of parathyroidectomy on quality of life and non-specific symptoms in normocalcaemic primary hyperparathyroidism. Br J Surg 2018;105(3):223–9.
11. Voss L, Nobrega M, Bandeira L, et al. Impaired physical function and evaluation of quality of life in normocalcemic and hypercalcemic primary hyperparathyroidism. Bone 2020;141:115583.
12. Rao DS, Phillips ER, Divine GW, et al. Randomized controlled clinical trial of surgery versus no surgery in patients with mild asymptomatic primary hyperparathyroidism. J Clin Endocrinol Metab 2004;89(11):5415–22.
13. Bollerslev J, Jansson S, Mollerup CL, et al. Medical observation, compared with parathyroidectomy, for asymptomatic primary hyperparathyroidism: a prospective, randomized trial. J Clin Endocrinol Metab 2007;92(5):1687–92.
14. Ambrogini E, Cetani F, Fau-Cianferotti L, et al. Surgery or surveillance for mild asymptomatic primary hyperparathyroidism: a prospective, randomized clinical trial. J Clin Endocrinol Metab 2007;92(8):3114–21.
15. Pretorius MA-O, Lundstam KA-O, Hellström M, et al. Effects of parathyroidectomy on quality of life: 10 years of data from a prospective randomized controlled trial on primary hyperparathyroidism (the SIPH-Study). J Bone Miner Res 2021;36(1):3–11.
16. Webb SM, Puig-Domingo M, Villabona C, et al. Validation of PHPQoL, a disease-specific quality-of-life questionnaire for patients with primary hyperparathyroidism. J Clin Endocrinol Metab 2016;101(4):1571–8.
17. Ryhanen EM, Heiskanen I, Sintonen H, et al. Health-related quality of life is impaired in primary hyperparathyroidism and significantly improves after surgery: a prospective study using the 15D instrument. Endocr Connect 2015;4(3):179–86.
18. Walker MD, McMahon DJ, Inabnet WB, et al. Neuropsychological features in primary hyperparathyroidism: a prospective study. J Clin Endocrinol Metab 2009;94(6):1951–8.
19. Roman SJ, Pietrzak RH, Snyder PJ, et al. The effects of serum calcium and parathyroid hormone changes on psychological and cognitive function in patients undergoing parathyroidectomy for primary hyperparathyroidism. Ann Surg 2011;253(1):131–7.

20. Espiritu RP Ka, Vickers ks, Grant c, et al. Depression in primary hyperparathyroidism: prevalence and benefit of surgery. J Clin Endocrinol Metab 2011; 96(11):E1737–45.
21. Liu JYPB, Mlaver E, Patel SG, et al. Neuropsychologic changes in primary hyperparathyroidism after parathyroidectomy from a dual-institution prospective study. Surgery 2021;169(1):114–9.
22. Pasieka JPL, Demeure MJ, Wilson S, et al. Patient-based Surgical Outcome Tool Demonstrating Alleviation of Symptoms following Parathyroidectomy in Patients with Primary Hyperparathyroidism. World J Surg 2002;26:942–9.
23. Weber TKM, Hense I, Pietsch A, et al. Effect of parathyroidectomy on quality of life and neuropsychological symptoms in primary hyperparathyroidism. World J Surg 2007;31:1202–9.
24. Brazier JEHR, Jones NM, O'Cathain A, et al. Validating the SF-36 health survey questionnaire: new outcome measure for primary care. Bmj 1992;18(305):160–4.
25. van Leeuwaarde RSPC, May AM, Dekkers OM, et al. Health-related quality of life in patients with multiple endocrine neoplasia type 1. Neuroendocrinology 2021; 111(3):288–96.
26. van der Meulen MZNA, Lobatto DJ, Andela CD, et al. SF-12 or SF-36 in pituitary disease? Toward concise and comprehensive patient-reported outcomes measurements. Endocrine 2020;70(1):123–33.
27. Ware JE Jr, Sherbourne CD. The MOS 36-item short-form health survey (SF-36). I. Conceptual framework and item selection. Med Care 1992;30(6):473–83.
28. Mihai RSG. Pasieka's parathyroid symptoms scores correlate with SF-36 scores in patients undergoing surgery for primary hyperparathyroidism. World J Surg 2008;32:807–14.
29. Webb SM, Puig-Domingo M, Villabona C, et al. Development of a new tool for assessing health-related quality of life in patients with primary hyperparathyroidism. Health Qual Life Outcomes 2013;11:97.
30. Sintonen H. The 15D instrument of health-related quality of life: properties and applications. Ann Med 2001;33:328–36.
31. Parks KAPC, Onwuameze OE, Shrestha S. Psychiatric complications of primary hyperparathyroidism and mild hypercalcemia. Am J Psychiatry 2017;17(7): 620–2.
32. Trombetti ACE, Henzen C, Gold G, et al. Clinical presentation and management of patients with primary hyperparathyroidism of the Swiss Primary Hyperparathyroidism Cohort: a focus on neuro-behavioral and cognitive symptoms. J Endocrinol Invest 2016;39(5):567–76.
33. Eufrazino C, Veras A, Bandeira F. Epidemiology of primary hyperparathyroidism and its non-classical manifestations in the city of recife, Brazil. Clin Med Ins 2013;6:69–74.
34. Liu MSM, Cong E, Colon I, et al. Cognition and cerebrovascular function in primary hyperparathyroidism before and after parathyroidectomy. J Endocrinol Invest 2020;43(3):369–79.
35. Yadav SK, Mishra SK, Mishra A, et al. Changing profile of primary hyperparathyroidism over two and half decades: A Study in Tertiary Referral Center of North India. World J Surg 2018;42(9):2732–7.
36. Prasarttong-Osoth PWP, Imruetaicharoenchoke W, Rojananin S. Primary hyperparathyroidism: 11-year experience in a single institute in Thailand. Int J Endocrinol 2012;2012:952426.
37. Cipriani C, Bilezikian JP. Three generational phenotypes of sporadic primary hyperparathyroidism: evolution defined by technology 2019;7(10):745–7.

38. Minisola S, Pepe J, Scillitani A, et al. Explaining geographical variation in the presentation of primary hyperparathyroidism. Lancet Diab Endocrinol 2016;4(8): 641–3.
39. Rolighed L, Amstrup AK, Jakobsen NF, et al. Muscle function is impaired in patients with "asymptomatic" primary hyperparathyroidism. World J Surg 2014; 38(3):549–57.
40. A° berg VNS, Zedenius J, Saa f M, et al. Health-related quality of life after successful surgery for primary hyperparathyroidism:no additive effect from vitamin D supplementation: results of a double-blind randomized study. Europ J Endocrinol 2015;172(2):181–7.
41. Bilezikian JP, Khan AA, Silverberg SJ, et al. Evaluation and Management of Primary Hyperparathyroidism: Summary Statement and Guidelines from the Fifth International Workshop. Available at: https://publons.com/publon/10.1002/jbmr.4677. Accessed August 19, 2022. DOI: https://doi.org/10.1002/jbmr.4677.
42. Bilezikian JP, Brandi ML, Eastell R, et al. Guidelines for the management of asymptomatic primary hyperparathyroidism: summary statement from the Fourth International Workshop. J Clin Endocrinol Metab 2014;99(10):3561–9.
43. Khan AA, Hanley DA, Rizzoli R, et al. Primary hyperparathyroidism: review and recommendations on evaluation, diagnosis, and management. a Canadian and international consensus. Osteoporos Int 2017;28(1):1–19.
44. Roman SASJ, Mayes L, Desmond E, et al. Parathyroidectomy improves neurocognitive deficits in patients with primary hyperparathyroidism. Surgery 2005; 138:1121–8.
45. Brito KES, Eslick GD. The extent of improvement of health-related quality of life as assessed by the SF36 and Paseika scales after parathyroidectomy in patients with primary hyperparathyroidism–a systematic review and meta-analysis. Int J Surg 2015;13:245–9.
46. Sheldon DGLF, Neil NJ, Ryan JA Jr. Surgical treatment of hyperparathyroidism improves health-related quality of life. Arch Surg 2002;137:1022–6.
47. Greutelaers BKK, Kollias J, Bochner M, et al. Pasieka Illness Questionnaire: its value in primary hyperparathyroidism. ANZ J Surg 2004;74:112–5.
48. Caillard CSF, Mathonnet M, Gibelin H, et al. Prospective evaluation of quality of life (SF-36v2) and nonspecific symptoms before and after cure of primary hyperparathyroidism (1-year follow-up). Surgery 2007;141:153–9.
49. Leong KJSR, Garnham AW. Health-related quality of life improvement following surgical treatment of primary hyperparathyroidism in a United Kingdom population. Surgeon 2010;8:5–8.
50. Ramakant PVA, Chand G, Mishra A, et al. Salutary effect of parathyroidectomy on neuropsychiatric symptoms in patients with primary hyperparathyroidism: evaluation using PAS and SF-36v2 scoring systems. J Postgrad Med 2011;57:96–101.
51. La JWT, Hammad AY, Burgardt L, et al. Parathyroidectomy for primary hyperparathyroidism improves sleep quality: a prospective study. Surgery 2017;161:25–34.
52. Tzikos GCA, Evangelos S, Boura E, et al. Quality of life in patients with asymptomatic primary hyperparathyroidism after parathyroidectomy: a 3-year longitudinal study. Endocr Pract 2021;27:716–22.
53. Pasieka JLPL, Jones J. The long-term benefit of parathyroidectomy in primary hyperparathyroidism: a 10-year prospective surgical outcome study. Surgery 2009; 146:1006–13.
54. Blanchard C, Mathonnet M, Sebag F, et al. Quality of life is modestly improved in older patients with mild primary hyperparathyroidism postoperatively: results of a prospective multicenter study. Ann Surg Oncol 2014;21(11):3534–40.

55. Dulfer RGW, Morks A, van Lieshout EM, et al. Impact of parathyroidectomy for primary hyperparathyroidism on quality of life: a case-control study using Short Form Health Survey 36. Head Neck 2016;38:1213–20.
56. Tolley NGG, Palazzo F, Prichard A, et al. Long-term prospective evaluation comparing robotic parathyroidectomy with minimally invasive open parathyroidectomy for primary hyperparathyroidism. Head Neck 2016;38(Suppl 1):E300–6.
57. Perrier NDBD, Wefel JS, Jimenez C, et al. Prospective, randomized, controlled trial of parathyroidectomy versus observation in patients with "asymptomatic" primary hyperparathyroidism. Surgery 2009;146:1116–22.
58. Morris GSGE, Hearon CM, Gantela S, et al. Parathyroidectomy improves functional capacity in "asymptomatic" older patients with primary hyperparathyroidism: a randomized control trial. Ann Surg 2010;251:832–7.
59. Anagnostis PVK, Veneti S, Potoupni V, et al. Efficacy of parathyroidectomy compared with active surveillance in patients with mild asymptomatic primary hyperparathyroidism: a systematic review and meta-analysis of randomized-controlled studies. J Endocrinol Invest 2021;44:1127–37.
60. Ejlsmark-Svensson HST, Webb SM, Rejnmark L, et al. Health-related quality of life improves 1 year after parathyroidectomy in primary hyperparathyroidism: A prospective cohort study. Clin Endocrinol 2019;90:184–91.
61. Walker MDSS. Quality of life in primary hyperparathyroidism revisited: keep calm and carry on? J Bone Miner Res 2021;36(1):1–2.
62. Ng CHCY, Tan MHQ, Ng JX, et al. Cinacalcet and primary hyperparathyroidism: systematic review and meta regression. Endocr Connect 2020;9:724–35.
63. Timmons JGMR, Bailey M, McDougall C. Cognitive impairment reversed by cinacalcet administration in primary hyperparathyroidism. Hormones 2021;20:587–9.
64. Koman ABR, Pernow Y, Bränström R, et al. Prediction of cognitive response to surgery in elderly patients with primary hyperparathyroidism. BJS Open 2021;5(2):zraa029.
65. Koman AOS, Bränström R, Pernow Y, et al. Short-term medical treatment of hypercalcaemia in primary hyperparathyroidism predicts symptomatic response after parathyroidectomy. BJS 2019;106:1810–8.
66. Singh Ospina N, Maraka S, Rodriguez-Gutierrez R, et al. Comparative efficacy of parathyroidectomy and active surveillance in patients with mild primary hyperparathyroidism: a systematic review and meta-analysis. Osteoporos Int 2016;27(12):3395–407.
67. Papavramidis TSAP, Pliakos I, Tzikos G, et al. The impact of age on quality of life and frailty outcomes after parathyroidectomy in patients with primary hyperparathyroidism. J Endocrinol Invest 2021;45(4):797–802.

UNITED STATES POSTAL SERVICE®

Statement of Ownership, Management, and Circulation (All Periodicals Publications Except Requester Publications)

1. Publication Title	2. Publication Number	3. Filing Date
ENDOCRINOLOGY AND METABOLISM CLINICS OF NORTH AMERICA	000 – 275	9/18/2022
4. Issue Frequency	5. Number of Issues Published Annually	6. Annual Subscription Price
MAR, JUN, SEP, DEC	4	$394.00

7. Complete Mailing Address of Known Office of Publication *(Not printer) (Street, city, county, state, and ZIP+4®)*
ELSEVIER INC.
230 Park Avenue, Suite 800
New York, NY 10169

Contact Person
Malathi Samayan
Telephone *(Include area code)*
91-44-4299-4507

8. Complete Mailing Address of Headquarters or General Business Office of Publisher *(Not printer)*
ELSEVIER INC.
230 Park Avenue, Suite 800
New York, NY 10169

9. Full Names and Complete Mailing Addresses of Publisher, Editor, and Managing Editor *(Do not leave blank)*

Publisher *(Name and complete mailing address)*
TAYLOR HAYES, ELSEVIER INC.
1600 JOHN F KENNEDY BLVD. SUITE 1800
PHILADELPHIA, PA 19103-2899

Editor *(Name and complete mailing address)*
KATERINA HEIDHAUSEN, ELSEVIER INC.
1600 JOHN F KENNEDY BLVD. SUITE 1800
PHILADELPHIA, PA 19103-2899

Managing Editor *(Name and complete mailing address)*
PATRICK MANLEY, ELSEVIER INC.
1600 JOHN F KENNEDY BLVD. SUITE 1800
PHILADELPHIA, PA 19103-2899

10. Owner *(Do not leave blank. If the publication is owned by a corporation, give the name and address of the corporation immediately followed by the names and addresses of all stockholders owning or holding 1 percent or more of the total amount of stock. If not owned by a corporation, give the names and addresses of the individual owners. If owned by a partnership or other unincorporated firm, give its name and address as well as those of each individual owner. If the publication is published by a nonprofit organization, give its name and address.)*

Full Name	Complete Mailing Address
WHOLLY OWNED SUBSIDIARY OF REED/ELSEVIER, US HOLDINGS	1600 JOHN F KENNEDY BLVD. SUITE 1800 PHILADELPHIA, PA 19103-2899

11. Known Bondholders, Mortgagees, and Other Security Holders Owning or Holding 1 Percent or More of Total Amount of Bonds, Mortgages, or Other Securities. If none, check box → ☐ None

Full Name	Complete Mailing Address
N/A	

12. Tax Status *(For completion by nonprofit organizations authorized to mail at nonprofit rates) (Check one)*
The purpose, function, and nonprofit status of this organization and the exempt status for federal income tax purposes:
☒ Has Not Changed During Preceding 12 Months
☐ Has Changed During Preceding 12 Months *(Publisher must submit explanation of change with this statement)*

13. Publication Title	14. Issue Date for Circulation Data Below
ENDOCRINOLOGY AND METABOLISM CLINICS OF NORTH AMERICA	JUNE 2022

15. Extent and Nature of Circulation			Average No. Copies Each Issue During Preceding 12 Months	No. Copies of Single Issue Published Nearest to Filing Date
a. Total Number of Copies *(Net press run)*			225	179
b. Paid Circulation *(By Mail and Outside the Mail)*	(1)	Mailed Outside-County Paid Subscriptions Stated on PS Form 3541 (Include paid distribution above nominal rate, advertiser's proof copies, and exchange copies)	103	84
	(2)	Mailed In-County Paid Subscriptions Stated on PS Form 3541 *(Include paid distribution above nominal rate, advertiser's proof copies, and exchange copies)*	0	0
	(3)	Paid Distribution Outside the Mails Including Sales Through Dealers and Carriers, Street Vendors, Counter Sales, and Other Paid Distribution Outside USPS®	71	60
	(4)	Paid Distribution by Other Classes of Mail Through the USPS (e.g., First-Class Mail®)	0	0
c. Total Paid Distribution *[Sum of 15b (1), (2), (3), and (4)]* ▶			174	144
d. Free or Nominal Rate Distribution *(By Mail and Outside the Mail)*	(1)	Free or Nominal Rate Outside-County Copies included on PS Form 3541	32	18
	(2)	Free or Nominal Rate In-County Copies Included on PS Form 3541	0	0
	(3)	Free or Nominal Rate Copies Mailed at Other Classes Through the USPS (e.g., First-Class Mail)	0	0
	(4)	Free or Nominal Rate Distribution Outside the Mail *(Carriers or other means)*	0	0
e. Total Free or Nominal Rate Distribution *(Sum of 15d (1), (2), (3) and (4))*			32	18
f. Total Distribution *(Sum of 15c and 15e)* ▶			206	162
g. Copies not Distributed *(See Instructions to Publishers #4 (page #3))* ▶			19	17
h. Total *(Sum of 15f and g)*			225	179
i. Percent Paid *(15c divided by 15f times 100)* ▶			84.46%	88.88%

* If you are claiming electronic copies, go to line 16 on page 3. If you are not claiming electronic copies, skip to line 17 on page 3.

16. Electronic Copy Circulation	Average No. Copies Each Issue During Preceding 12 Months	No. Copies of Single Issue Published Nearest to Filing Date
a. Paid Electronic Copies ▶		
b. Total Paid Print Copies (Line 15c) + Paid Electronic Copies (Line 16a) ▶		
c. Total Print Distribution (Line 15f) + Paid Electronic Copies (Line 16a) ▶		
d. Percent Paid (Both Print & Electronic Copies) (16b divided by 16c × 100) ▶		

☒ **I certify that 50% of all my distributed copies (electronic and print) are paid above a nominal price.**

17. Publication of Statement of Ownership
☒ If the publication is a general publication, publication of this statement is required. Will be printed in the DECEMBER 2022 issue of this publication. ☐ Publication not required.

18. Signature and Title of Editor, Publisher, Business Manager, or Owner
Malathi Samayan - Distribution Controller — *Malathi Samayan* — Date: 9/18/2022

I certify that all information furnished on this form is true and complete. I understand that anyone who furnishes false or misleading information on this form or who omits material or information requested on the form may be subject to criminal sanctions (including fines and imprisonment) and/or civil sanctions (including civil penalties).

Printed and bound by CPI Group (UK) Ltd, Croydon, CR0 4YY
08/05/2025
01864719-0003